SPECIALIZATION AND CREDENTIALING IN NURSING REVISITED:

UNDERSTANDING THE ISSUES, ADVANCING THE PROFESSION

Margretta Madden Styles, EdD, RN, FAAN
Mary Jean Schumann, RN, MSN, MBA, CPNP
Carol J. Bickford, PhD, RN-BC
Kathleen White, PhD, RN, CNAA-BC

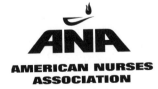

AMERICAN NURSES ASSOCIATION

SILVER SPRING, MARYLAND
2008

Library of Congress Cataloging-in-Publication Data

Styles, Margretta M.

Specialization and credentialing in nursing revisited : understanding the issues, advancing the profession / Margretta Madden Styles . . . [et al.].

p. ; cm.

Includes bibliographical references and index.

ISBN-13: 978-1-55810-257-6 (pbk.)

ISBN-10: 1-55810-257-4 (pbk.)

1. Nursing specialties. I. Styles, Margretta M. II. American Nurses Association.

[DNLM: 1. Specialties, Nursing—standards. 2. Credentialing—standards. WY 101 S741 2008]

RT86.7.S78 2008

610.73—dc22

2008004470

The American Nurses Association (ANA) is a national professional association. This ANA publication—*Specialization and Credentialing In Nursing Revisited: Understanding The Issues, Advancing The Profession*—reflects thoughts developed by independent authors in response to the ANA's call for writers on various topics within the practice of nursing. This publication should be reviewed in conjunction with state board of nursing policies and practices. State laws, rules, and regulations govern the practice of nursing, while *Specialization and Credentialing In Nursing Revisited: Understanding The Issues, Advancing The Profession*, guides nurses in the application of their professional skills and responsibilities. The information in this book should not be interpreted as legal or professional advice.

ANA is the only full-service professional organization representing the nation's 2.9 million Registered Nurses through its 54 constituent member associations. ANA advances the nursing profession by fostering high standards of nursing practice, promoting the economic and general welfare of nurses in the workplace, projecting a positive and realistic view of nursing, and lobbying the Congress and regulatory agencies on health-care issues affecting nurses and the public.

Published by Nursesbooks.org
The Publishing Program of ANA
American Nurses Association
8515 Georgia Avenue, Suite 400
Silver Spring, MD 20910-3492
1-800-274-4ANA
http://www.Nursesbooks.org/

Design and Composition:
House of Equations, Inc., Arden, NC
Stacy Maguire, Sterling, VA
Editing:
Steven A. Jent, Denton, TX
Lisa Munsat Anthony, Chapel Hill, NC
Ashley Mason, Atlanta, GA
Printing:
McArdle Printing, Upper Marlboro, MD

ISBN-13: 978-55810-257-6   SAN: 851-3481   2.5M   04/08

First printing April 2008.

CONTENTS

Chapter 5. Afterthoughts on a Styles Scenario
Margretta Madden Styles

ABOUT THE AUTHORS

Margretta (Gretta) Madden Styles, EdD, RN, FAAN (1930–2006), had extensive national and international experience in nursing education and credentialing. She was professor and dean of nursing schools at the University of California, San Francisco; Wayne State University; and the University of Texas Health Science Center, San Antonio.

Gretta chaired the ANA National Study of Credentialing in Nursing (1979). In 1983 the American Nurses' Foundation (ANF) named her its first Distinguished Scholar. In this capacity she studied the movement toward specialization in nursing and published *On Specialization in Nursing: Toward a New Empowerment* in 1989. As a result of its recommendation for creation of a board of specialties, the support of the Macy Foundation, and the diligence of many nurse leaders, the American Board of Nursing Specialties was established in 1991.

While president of ANA from 1986 to 1988 and chair of the Commission on Organizational Assessment and Renewal (COAR), Gretta was instrumental in the establishment of the American Nurses Credentialing Center (ANCC). She was president of ANCC from 1996 to 1998. At the state level, she was a member and president of the California Board of Registered Nursing (1992–93).

As consultant to the International Council of Nurses (ICN), Gretta authored the organization's position on nursing regulation (1985) and participated in regional workshops on nursing regulation around the world. In Geneva she also chaired a World Health Organization (WHO) advisory group on nursing regulation. Dr. Styles served as ICN's president from 1993 until 1997. Largely for her global work in credentialing, she was awarded the 2005 ICN Christiane Reimann Prize.

Mary Jean Schumann, RN, MSN, MBA, CPNP, is Director, Nursing Practice and Policy, American Nurses Association where she oversees national practice and policy issues related to advanced practice registered nurses. In addition, her department provides for the national work relative to nursing scopes and standards of practice, the International Council of Nurses, nursing shortage and staffing issues, nursing quality, the National Database of Nursing Quality Indicators, nursing informatics, electronic health records and Nurse Competence in Aging. Ms. Schumann also provides the oversight to ANA's Congress of Nursing Practice and Economics. She has been a nationally certified pediatric nurse practitioner since 1984, past Executive Director of the national Pediatric Nursing Certification Board (PNCB), and has been active in addressing issues of infant mental health, adolescent pregnancy prevention and parenting, and college health, and in the provision of hospice services. Ms. Schumann was a 1991–1993 Commonwealth Fund Fellow.

Carol J. Bickford, PhD, RN-BC, provides direction and support for the American Nurses Association's informatics and professional practice and standards initiatives and committees in her role as Senior Policy Fellow in the Department of Nursing Practice and Policy. She serves as ANA's staff resource person to the nursing scope and standards work both internally and externally to many national speciality nursing organizations. She also represents nurses and ANA at numerous national tables on informatics, electronic health records, the documentation of health care, and nursing languages and terminologies.

Kathleen M. White, PhD, RN, CNAA,BC is an Associate Professor at The Johns Hopkins University, School of Nursing, where she is the Director of the Masters' Program and Interim Director of the Doctor of Nursing Practice Program. Dr. White is currently the Chairperson for the American Nurses Association Congress on Nursing Practice and Economics and served from 1999–2006 on the ANA Committee on Nursing Practice Standards and Guidelines. Under her leadership the 2004 version of the scope and standards for nursing practice were written and became the standards that define the practice and professional role expectations for all nurses in the United States. Kathleen is also a member of the Board of Directors of Carefirst Blue Cross and Blue Shield; Chairperson for the Maryland Patient Safety Center Board of Directors; and a member of the Maryland Health Care Commission's Hospital Performance Evaluation Guide Advisory Committee.

FOREWORD

This book carries a heavy burden: it frames the recent history of the complex issue of specialization, subspecialization, and credentialing in nursing at the advanced practice level. Describing the lack of a shared framework among and between the various professional bodies charged with the stewardship of the profession, it offers a unity model and pathway the profession might follow to create a consistent and supported methodology to define specialty and subspecialty practice, and it issues a call to action. Indeed, it's a lot for one small book.

It is clear the profession is not in agreement as to the definition and scope of specialty and subspecialty practice. Nor is there agreement as to the need for shared core competencies among various areas of advanced practice. There has been a proliferation of advanced practice curriculums as well as certification examinations focused on highly specialized areas of practice and the competing desire on the part of regulators, sometimes at the state level, to limit access to advanced practice to those with broad academic preparation, which is age-specific. Such positions have been vigorously challenged by nursing associations, colleges of nursing, faculty organizations, and others.

The lack of a mutually agreed-upon paradigm has allowed the proliferation of an ever growing number of approaches to specialty and subspecialty practice and has left advanced practitioners vulnerable in a number of ways; third party reimbursement and license portability are just two examples. Successful completion of an academic program and the subsequent passing of various specialty certification examinations is no longer a guarantee that one may practice in one's chosen area from one state to another as various state boards of nursing define advanced specialty practice differently.

The lack of a unifying model has brought us to the brink of chaos, exposed the profession to challenge, and placed our advanced practitioners in a most difficult position. It is impossible, under these circumstances to envision an empowered practice environment. Thus a call to action is framed in the last chapters of this book. We must agree to one paradigm for specialty and subspecialty practice if full empowerment is to be realized.

The lead author of this book, Margretta Madden Styles, spent much of her career framing and outlining specialty practice. Gretta had just completed her work for this book when, sadly, she succumbed to her final illness. She believed passionately that specialty practice, especially at the advanced practice level, would lead nursing into the future. She spent much of the later part of her career framing, refining, and defining the components of specialty practice not only for nursing in the United States but around the world. She leaves us with a model and a process by which to define specialty and subspecialty practice. She challenges us to find consensus and rally around a model. Those of us who knew Gretta should not be surprised that she has done so.

Mary Jean Schumann, Kathi White, and Carol Bickford, have each provided clear insight into the issues surrounding specialty and subspecialty practice as well as framing the historical issues that influence today's reality. The profession is well served here.

This book envisions a future, frames a process, and issues a challenge. Together we must put our house in order. To do anything less is unthinkable.

Barbara A. Blakeney, MS, RN
Immediate Past President,
American Nurses Association (2002–2006)
The Center for Innovations in Care Delivery
The Institute of Patient Care
Massachusetts General Hospital
Boston, Massachusetts

Background information

In December of 2004 the American Nurses Association, in partnership with the American College of Nursing sponsored a conference of advanced practice nursing stakeholders at its headquarters in Silver Spring, Maryland. ANA President Barbara Blakeney opened that meeting with the charge to the assembled group that the goal must be agreement as to the process by which specialty and subspecialty practice at the advanced practice level be defined. The meeting was to begin the process of finding a model—a framework that would allow the work to proceed. Because of her ground-breaking work on specialty practice, Dr. Margretta Madden Styles was invited to present the history of specialty practice and to suggest a framework through which the work could be accomplished. The text of the slides of her presentation are reproduced in Appendix B.

PREFACE

In 1989, mid-way in my "credentialing career," my book *On Specialization in Nursing: Toward a New Empowerment**, was published by the American Nurses Foundation. It began with a biological metaphor applying natural laws to the development of the professional organism. It depicted specialization as a process and nursing as an evolving social system. It analyzed a survey of specialties and graduate programs existing at that time, and it identified some uncertainties and inconsistencies that might undermine the specialization movement. It set forth economic, social, and practice indices of professional empowerment and discussed their relation to the power of specialty credentials at that time.

Finally, it offered a number of proposals for empowering nursing as an evolving and specialized profession:

▌ The essentials of empowerment
▌ A mechanism and criteria for approving specialties (the basis for the formation of the American Board of Nursing Specialties)
▌ Steps to accomplish these goals

The study and its recommendations did not substantially address the advanced practice movement, then early in its development.

Now is the time for another look. In the last 20 years the situation has changed dramatically, influenced by a number of forces. Specialties have continued to proliferate and become more narrow. Conceptual and practical debates about specialties and subspecialties on both basic and advanced practice levels are heating up and becoming more confounding. Questions and challenges arise as to what are appropriate credentials and what scope of practice and privileges should be associated with

_____

* The primary text of that 1989 book is reproduced in this volume as Appendix C.

them. The respective and complementary roles of credentialing agents have become more confusing. Mismatches between graduate curricula and requirements for certification and licensing sometimes leave graduates caught in the middle.

We must reach agreement on these fundamental questions, or the whole system may collapse. As a profession we must accept responsibility for the problems and accountability for the solutions. These are matters for us to settle internally. Our decisions will prevail in the external environment if we present them in unity and with clarity and reason.

Gretta Styles, 2005

Introduction: Why Revisit Nursing Regulation?

Twice in the last dozen years a critically divisive issue has caused heated debate in the advanced practice registered nurse community. The issue: what level of nursing practice fits the education and credentials of the individual nurse? This debate has involved major accrediting organizations, certifying bodies, state boards of nursing, professional nursing organizations, and thousands of registered nurses (RNs) and advanced practice registered nurses (APRNs).

The debate has its roots in the continuing evolution of nursing practice. Similarly, the emergence of dozens of specialized nursing practices has prompted challenges to nurses' expertise in caring for any given patient population.

Dr. Styles, in her 1989 book on specialization in nursing, discussed the development of specialization and what it has meant to the profession. She also described in detail how specialized knowledge and skills were recognized at that time, through mechanisms that included criteria for recognition of a nursing specialty, peer review for specialty organizations, and voluntary specialty certification of individuals. (The primary text of that 1989 book is reproduced in Appendix C.)

The trends in specialization did not occur just at the level of the generic nurse with a Bachelor of Science in Nursing (BSN) degree. Specialization led to the advanced practice roles of nurse practitioners, clinical nurse specialists, nurse midwives, and nurse anesthetists. These roles demanded more advanced knowledge and education beyond the BSN. Initially, with the exception of clinical nurse specialist programs, many of the advanced practice educational curricula were certificate programs not leading to a master's degree. However, by the early 1990s most certificate programs had been replaced by master's degree programs and the newer certificate, if there was one, was a post-master's certificate.

The impact of this trend toward greater specialization and the concomitant need for advanced education might not have caused such controversy if advanced practice nursing had either remained at a low level of acceptance or otherwise remained below the radar screen where it did not prompt additional scrutiny by those outside the profession.

Specialization and Credentialing in Nursing Revisited: Understanding the Issues, Advancing the Profession serves to clarify for all parties the current status of accreditation, educational standards, certification, and regulation, especially for advanced practice nursing. Such an overview needs to record not only the history, but also to describe the current scope and standards of practice along a single continuum as well as the safeguards in place to ensure safe and competent advanced practice registered nurses. This knowledge of these improvements will inform those who attempt to resolve what they perceive as conflicting approaches to APRN regulation. The book is organized as summarized below:

- Chapter 1 covers current events relating to specialty nursing practice, both basic and advanced. Included are descriptions of today's professional practice environment, progress in the advanced nursing practice arena, the latest definition of nursing, and the evolution of the nursing scope and standards of practice.
- Chapter 2 presents Dr. Styles' perspective on critical events within the advanced practice nursing movement in the 21st century, with an emphasis on the roles and influence of credentialing and credentialing agencies. In many ways advanced practice is at the cutting edge of nursing's ongoing struggle for professional status. Thus advanced practice issues are formative issues—that is, so fundamental to the evolution of the profession, its social contribution, and its future. The decisions to be made and the actions to be taken are key steps in building the profession. How nursing proceeds will reflect the current values of the profession.
- Chapter 3 provides an update on the current roles of APRNs and the conflicting views of how they should be regulated. It discusses the impact of further specialization on accreditation, education, credentialing and regulation of APRNs, including the latest efforts to create a less confusing methodology for those who regulate or choose to be regulated. Also provided are recent facts and figures about numbers of advanced practice specialties, numbers of APRNs, requirements for qualification, programs preparing APRNs, certifying bodies, state board and multi-state provisions for APRNs, accreditation and recognition of certifying bodies, and accreditation of educational programs.
- Chapter 4, also by Dr. Styles, first proposes principles underlying a prototype system for APRNs, in the interest of the public and the profession. A series of models follows, ranging from the generic to the highly specialized. The discussion stresses the essential nature of the processes utilized in applying the principles and determining the APRN model to be implemented. The underlying thesis is that only through reaching and fulfilling professional *accord* can nursing build this essential pillar of our practice.
- Chapter 5 conveys Dr. Styles's thoughts on a future-oriented, purely generic model for the profession, with all nurses educated at the graduate level. It rep-

resents her belief that the APRN movement will be the greatest impetus toward that goal, particularly in a more role-focused model of regulation.

Three appendixes supplement this primary material:

- Appendix A provides a data table that reflects the current depth and breadth of APRN preparation as of January 1, 2007, the latest for which reliable data was available.
- Appendix B reproduces Dr. Styles's *Address to the National Nurses Stakeholder Meeting on Advanced Practice* (December 16, 2004 in slide format).
- Appendix C is a reprint of the main text of the 1989 publication *On Specialization in Nursing: Toward a New Empowerment* by Gretta Styles.

In the original edition, all facts, figures, issues, and developments are from the 1980s, serving as a baseline for measuring how the situation has changed and how it has not. The frameworks for problem analysis and for examining the relative power of specialty credentials remain useful today.

The first edition of Dr. Styles' work is included at the back of this book to better allow the reader the perspective of the past at different points along the way in the development of the APRN. Understanding this part of nursing's recent history may assist the reader, much in the manner of a case study, to see a clearer path to the future.

What were the goals and recommendations then? Has the profession made progress toward achieving them? Schemes for organizing specialties and subspecialties were presented. In particular, the American Board of Nursing Specialties, first proposed therein, has made remarkable progress. It would be of historical interest to investigate to what extent nursing has followed, diverged from, or gone beyond the specialization concept as presented by Dr. Styles.

The authors hope that this new volume, in revisiting a critical issue for the nursing profession, provides multiple perspectives about specialization and credentialing in nursing and in the advanced practice of registered nurses.

Mary Jean Schumann
March 2008

Chapter 1

Specialty Nursing Practice in Today's World

Kathleen White, PhD, RN, CNAA-BC
and Carol J. Bickford, PhD, RN-BC

Over the past two decades much has changed for nursing, but some things remain constant. The four domains of practice, administration, education, and research continue as the areas of focus for the majority of registered nurses. The boundaries of these domains still overlap and expand as both healthcare settings and practice evolve.

Today's Environment

The American Nurses Association (ANA), the professional association for all nurses, continues its advocacy for the baccalaureate as the entry-level degree in nursing. In 2005 the American Organization of Nurse Executives (AONE) announced its position on practice and educational partnerships for the future, which specified that the nurse of the future should be educated at the baccalaureate level. Diploma schools of nursing have essentially disappeared as a primary source for the preparation of applicants to sit for the nursing licensure exam, NCLEX, and assume the title of Registered Nurse (RN). Community colleges have established associate degree programs for registered nurses and continue to be the largest provider of new RNs, preparing 42.2% versus 31% from baccalaureate programs (HRSA 2004; http://bhpr.hrsa.gov/healthworkforce/reports/rnpopulation/preliminaryfindings.htm).

Entry into practice for registered nurses now includes additional options that were unavailable to individuals interested in this profession in the mid-1980s. Educational institutions have created RN preparation tracks for students who have already completed a practical nurse or vocational nurse program and are licensed at that level. Increasing numbers of applicants now seek admission to nursing programs after completion of undergraduate and even graduate degree programs in other fields. Additionally, students may enter nursing school and complete a generic master's degree (graduate entry pre-specialty in nursing) or a clinical nurse leader program as their entry level into nursing. Students may also find their way to completion of registered nursing programs through online programs of uneven quality and accreditation status.

The National Sample Survey of Registered Nurses

The graying of America's population is reflected in America's nurses. In 2004 only 8% of RNs were under age 30, the average age of RNs was 46.8 years, and over 41% of RNs were 50 years of age or older, according to the National Sample Survey of Registered Nurses (HRSA 2004; http://bhpr.hrsa.gov/healthworkforce/reports/rnpopulation/preliminaryfindings.htm). Similarly the National Student Nurses Association reports that only 32% of its membership is between the ages of 18 and 22 years (NSNA 2007; http://www.nsna.org/membership/pdf/faq.pdf).

The National Sample Survey of Registered Nurses is conducted by the Bureau of Health Professions every four years to profile the demographics, educational preparation, practice settings, and other pertinent workforce characteristics of registered nurses. Because of the increased interest, the 2004 survey included additional questions to explore specialty and advanced practice. In 2004 the number of APRNs (advanced practice registered nurses) was 240,460 (8.3% of all RNs); 70.1% of APRNs were certified, and 61.8% were recognized in one or more states as APRNs. There were 141,209 nurse practitioners, 72,521 clinical nurse specialists, 14,689 dually prepared as nurse practitioners and clinical nurse specialists, 32,523 certified registered nurse anesthetists (CRNAs), and 13,684 certified nurse midwives (CNMs).

In the 1980s Dr. Styles completed an environmental scan as part of her research into identifying the preparation for specialty nursing practice. At that time, preparation for specialty nursing practice was not formal master's preparation for an APRN role; it tended to be a result of on-the-job experiences, participation in continuing education, and self study. The success and recognition of APRN roles forced the creation of APRN educational curricula. Certification programs fostered new formal mechanisms to prepare for and recognize specialty practice at more advanced levels.

While clinical nurse specialists had from the conception of the role been educated only in master's degree programs, each of the other three categories—nurse midwives, nurse anesthetists, and nurse practitioners—had developed their roles through various levels of education. By the mid-1980s many of these programs were being taught in master's level curricula, yet this minimum requirement was not standardized.

Independent decision making and autonomy for these healthcare professionals in their practice roles and environments was becoming more widely accepted in some states. Many APRNs fought diligently for those rights, as well as for third-party reimbursement and prescriptive authority, in their states. Major long-term initiatives in the late 1980s resulted in further refinement of the APRN roles and the partial integration of these clinicians into mainstream healthcare practice and the reimbursement structures of Medicare, Medicaid, and other payers.

Over the last 20 years, the widespread acceptance of managed health care has challenged physicians' income, causing organized medicine to renew its pressure on APRNs in competition for a smaller revenue base. Suddenly the Medicaid payments that had seemed paltry to physician practices in the 1970s became an important factor in the continuing battles for APRNs' recognition and parity. In many cases, physician colleagues who had accepted APRNs as a valuable source of services withdrew their support in search of the redistribution of scarce healthcare dollars.

But not every registered nurse chooses to become an APRN when progressing from novice to expert clinician. Proponents of adequate preparation for specialty nursing practice must consider these individuals and their needs when defining specialty practice professional development programs in academic and continuing education settings. Today's increasingly complex healthcare environment has also prompted development of specialty nursing practice in non-clinical areas such as administration, case management, and informatics. Certification programs and advanced educational programs have been or are being created for these nursing specialty areas as well. Recently the American Association of Colleges of Nursing (AACN) established a road map and essentials for the doctorate of nursing practice (DNP), establishing the DNP as the educational preparation for all APRNs by 2015.

The ANA, after national discussions and deliberations with specialty nursing organizations about the characteristics of a nursing specialty, established a formal recognition program for new nursing specialties in the 1990s. The Congress on Nursing Practice and Economics (CNPE) oversees this program and acts on recommendations from its Committee on Nursing Practice Standards and Guidelines to recognize a nursing specialty, approve its scope of practice statement, and acknowledge specialty nursing standards of practice. A nursing specialty:

1. Defines itself as nursing;
2. Adheres to the overall licensure requirements of the profession;
3. Subscribes to the overall purposes and functions of nursing;
4. Is clearly defined;
5. Is practiced nationally or internationally;
6. Includes a substantial number of nurses who devote most of their practice to the specialty;
7. Can identify a need and demand for itself;
8. Has a well derived knowledge base particular to the practice of the nursing specialty;
9. Is concerned with phenomena of the discipline of nursing;
10. Defines competencies for the area of nursing specialty practice;
11. Has existing mechanisms for supporting, reviewing, and disseminating research to support its knowledge base;
12. Has defined educational criteria for specialty preparation or graduate degree;
13. Has continuing education programs or continuing competence mechanisms for nurses in the specialty; and
14. Is organized and represented by a national specialty association or branch of a parent organization.

Scope and Standards of Practice

In 2002 the American Nurses Association, in its continued role and ongoing responsibilities as the professional nursing organization, convened a work group as part of its regular review cycle of foundational documents to examine and, if necessary, revise the definition of nursing, scope of nursing practice statement, and standards of nursing practice. The work group was tasked to carefully review the current practice environment, existing nursing and specialty nursing scope and standards documents, and other materials and resources to identify the best mechanism to describe contemporary nursing practice and a framework for practice for the next five to ten years.

The work group's deliberations over two years resulted in a new definition of nursing, articulation of one scope of nursing practice, and standards of nursing practice with associated measurement criteria *applicable to all nurses*. The new standards of nursing practice also included additional measurement criteria for those in APRN and nursing role specialty practice, and they incorporated specific standards and measurement criteria applicable to APRN practice for consultation and prescriptive authority and treatment.

Nursing: Scope and Standards of Practice was published in 2004 after an extended field review and public comment period, subsequent revisions, review and revision by the ANA Committee on Nursing Practice Standards and Guidelines, and final review, revision, and approval by the ANA CNPE. Faculty members have integrated this content into academic and nursing professional development curricula. Nursing service departments use the standards and measurement criteria for position descriptions, performance evaluations, and the development of policy and procedures. This template language is now used by specialty nursing organizations to draft specialty nursing scope and standards of practice. Those facilities seeking American Nursing Credentialing Center (ANCC) Magnet™ recognition must incorporate such standards into practice, particularly the *Scope and Standards for Nurse Administrators* (ANA 2004b). Regulatory bodies, especially state boards of nursing, are encouraged to incorporate the content in their decision-making activities.

Chronology of Key Events

The current professional nursing environment is made up of many independent organizational structures driven by specialty practice.

Specialty Nursing Organizations

A group of specialty organizations established the National Federation of Specialty Nursing Organizations (NFSNO) in 1973 to address practice and leadership issues associated with specialty nursing. Through the 1970s more specialty nursing organizations emerged to address special interests and evolving practice. In 1982 ANA established the Nursing Organizations Liaison Forum (NOLF) to provide a forum for discussion and concerted action on professional policy and national health policy issues. It is not surprising that many specialty organizations belonged to both groups. ANA also maintained councils, committees, and special interest groups related to specialty practice interests.

In 2001 after years of duplicated effort, joint meetings, and then focused deliberations and negotiations, NFSNO and NOLF voted to create the Nursing Organizations Alliance (the Alliance). That action resulted in the dissolution of NFSNO and an ANA bylaws revision to close NOLF. Alliance membership is open to any nursing organization dedicated to current and emerging nursing and healthcare issues. Structural nursing components of a multidisciplinary organization are also welcome to join. Prior to this time, ANA had similarly restructured and divested itself of specialty practice councils and special interest groups (SIGs).

Credentialing and Certification for Specialty Practice

This evolution into separate, independent organizations similarly affected other sectors. As credentialing became an important component of the concept of quality practice, ANA's credentialing arm became a distinct and independent entity to prevent any conflict of interest issues. The **American Nurses Credentialing Center** (ANCC) was formed in 1991 as a corporation and subsidiary of ANA. Currently over 150,000 nurses in the United States and its territories carry ANCC certification as a credential in 40 specialty and advanced practice areas of nursing. ANCC holds accreditation from the National Commission for Certifying Agencies (NCCA) and the American Board of Nursing Specialties (ABNS).

The **National Commission for Certifying Agencies** (NCCA) is the accreditation body of the National Organization for Competency Assurance (NOCA), the leader in setting quality standards for credentialing organizations. Certification programs may apply to and be accredited by NCCA if they demonstrate compliance with all accreditation standards, standards that exceed the requirements set by the American Psychological Association and the U.S. Equal Employment Opportunity Commission (NCCA 2007; http://www.noca.org/Resources/NCCAAccreditation/tabid/82/Default.aspx).

The **American Board of Nursing Specialties** (ABNS) is a not-for-profit organization incorporated in 1991 after three years of dialogue within the nursing community to create uniformity in nursing certification and to increase public awareness of the value of quality certification to health care. ABNS advocates for consumer protection by establishing specialty nursing certification, and it represents over a half million certified registered nurses around the world through its member organizations (ABNS 2004; http://www.nursingcertification.org/pdf/Standards-revised-10-04.pdf).

Certification, as defined by ABNS, is the formal recognition of the specialized knowledge, skills, and experience demonstrated by the achievement of standards identified by a nursing specialty to promote optimal health outcomes. Individuals earn this credential after meeting defined criteria.

Accreditation is broadly defined as a voluntary, self-regulatory process by which governmental, non-governmental, or voluntary associations or other statutory bodies grant formal recognition to programs or institutions that meet stated quality criteria. For example, ABNS accreditation is a peer-reviewed process designed to protect the public interest by applying specific standards to the quality of nursing specialty certification examinations.

Regulation and Licensure

Nearly 100 years ago, boards of nursing were begun by state governments to protect the health of the public by overseeing and ensuring the safe practice of nursing. Individual state legislative bodies have charged their respective boards of nursing with the responsibility to protect the public through the regulation of individual licensed nurses, including registered nurses (RNs), licensed practical/vocational nurses (LPN/VNs), and advanced practice registered nurses (APRNs). By establishing a broad regulatory definition of nursing, boards of nursing can accommodate the changing healthcare environment, changing practice expectations, and the evolution of the profession. "Nursing Practice Acts and Nursing Administrative Rules/Regulations apply to all nursing roles in all settings. However, the regulatory definition of nursing practice needs to be specific enough to distinguish nursing practice from the practice of other health care practitioners" (NCSBN 2007b; https://www.ncsbn.org/156.htm).

The **National Council of State Boards of Nursing** (NCSBN) has a long and evolving history. It first began in 1932 as the Conference of State Boards of Nursing. At the request of state boards of nursing, ANA established a permanent Bureau of State Boards of Nursing in 1943. In a process of further evolution, ANA appointed a committee composed of one nurse representative from each state board of nursing, which was approved by the ANA Board of Directors in 1949 as the ANA Committee of State Boards of Nursing, and later became known as the ANA Council of State Boards of Nursing. This council voted to establish a separate autonomous nonprofit body, the National Council of State Boards of Nursing, Inc., in 1978. This entity, most often referred to as NCSBN, promotes discussion and unified action by the state boards of nursing "on matters of common interest and concern affecting public health, safety and welfare, which includes the development of licensure examinations for nursing."

NCSBN has coordinated the development of the multi-state RN compact for registered nurses to allow a nurse to be licensed in the state of residency and to practice in other states unless otherwise restricted. At this time only 23 state boards of nursing have elected to join the multi-state RN compact. More recently NCSBN created the Advanced Practice Compact, but this has received little support from state boards of nursing because of the far more complex and less standardized rules governing advanced practice from state to state (NCSBN 2007a; https://www.ncsbn.org/index.htm). NCSBN has also provided model nurse practice act language and guidance for individual state boards of nursing as they consider recognition of new nursing specialties.

Nursing Education and Specialization

The **American Association of Colleges of Nursing** (AACN) is a national organization for university and four-year college education programs in nursing, representing over 550 member schools. The mission of AACN is to establish quality standards for baccalaureate and graduate nursing education, assist deans and directors in implementing those standards, influence the nursing profession to improve health care, and promote public support of baccalaureate and graduate nursing education, research, and practice. AACN has an accreditation arm, the Commission on Collegiate Nursing Education (CCNE). Established in 1996, CCNE functions as an autonomous arm of AACN devoted exclusively to accreditation of baccalaureate and graduate nursing education programs. In 2000 CCNE was recognized as an accrediting organization by the U.S. Department of Education.

In its quest to standardize education, AACN has formed task forces to identify the essential elements of each level of education for the registered nurse. In order to be inclusive, these task forces have held regional meetings seeking input for the development of consensus-based standards documents from schools of nursing and stakeholders from various nursing organizations, regulatory boards, and practice settings.

The Essentials of Baccalaureate Education for Professional Nursing Practice (AACN 1998; http://www.aacn.nche.edu/Education/pdf/BaccEssentials98.pdf) is a comprehensive revision of the original standards for baccalaureate nursing released in 1986. It focuses on educating entry-level RNs and preparing professional nurses for practice in the twenty-first century. AACN has defined the "professional nurse" as an "individual prepared with a minimum of a baccalaureate in nursing but is inclusive of one who enters professional practice with a master's degree in nursing or a nursing doctorate." *Essentials* discusses both the discipline and the role of nursing. It delineates several components essential for all baccalaureate nursing programs for generalist level practice: liberal education, professional values, core competencies, core knowledge, and role development. An AACN task force convened to revise the *Essentials* document has completed the first draft, which outlines the expected competencies of graduates of baccalaureate nursing programs. Comments to this draft document are currently being received at regional meetings. The task force hopes to complete the revision by July 2008 for review and potential approval by the AACN Board of Directors at the 2008 board meeting. Approval of the membership would be sought at the October 2008 annual meeting.

The Essentials of Master's Education for Advanced Practice Nursing (AACN 1996; http://www.aacn.nche.edu/Education/pdf/MasEssentials96.pdf) was re-endorsed by the AACN Board of Directors in September 2004 without revision. It provides a three-part model for a Master's in Nursing curriculum:

1. The graduate nursing core—the foundational curriculum content necessary for all Master's students regardless of specialty or role

2. The advanced practice nursing core—essential content to provide direct patient or client services
3. The specialty curriculum content—that learning defined by the specialty organizations in order to care for a specialized patient or client

Master's Essentials further defines the graduate nursing curriculum core as including seven areas: research; policy, organization, and financing of health care; ethics; professional role development; theoretical foundations of nursing practice; human diversity and social issues; and health promotion and disease prevention. The advanced practice nursing core curriculum includes: advanced health and physical assessment, advanced physiology and pathophysiology, and advanced pharmacology.

However, the document does not define the nursing specialty curriculum nor the numbers of hours and types of clinical experiences required of graduates. The AACN suggests that each APRN organization, for instance the American College of Nurse-Midwives (ACNM), the American Association of Nurse Anesthetists (AANA), the National Association of Clinical Nurse Specialists (NACNS), and the National Organization of Nurse Practitioner Faculty (NONPF) define the curriculum and competencies for the specialty practice and the specific numbers of clinical hours and types of clinical experiences required for each. AACN states that it "endorses the minimum requirements defined by the specialty organizations for the individual APRN roles," further explaining that both the complexity of the specialty content as well as the need for adequate clinical exposure to develop the needed skills must be considered (AACN 1996, p.15; http://www.aacn.nche.edu/Education/pdf/MasEssentials96.pdf).

AACN published *Indicators of Quality in Research-focused Doctoral Programs in Nursing* in 2001 (http://www.aacn.nche.edu/publications/positions/qualityindicators.htm). This document acknowledges that although there are differences in purpose and curricula of doctor of philosophy (PhD) and doctor of nursing science (DNS) programs, most emphasize preparation for research. Therefore, AACN recommends continuing with a single set of quality indicators for research-focused doctoral programs in nursing, whether the program leads to a PhD or DNS degree. The recommended common elements of a program of study include: core and related course content including historical and philosophical foundations of nursing knowledge; existing and evolving substantive nursing knowledge; methods and processes of theory and knowledge development; research methods and scholarship appropriate to inquiry; and development related to roles in academic, research, practice, or policy environments. The teaching and learning should focus on progressive and guided experiences, with socialization and immersion to foster the student's development as a researcher in a specialty area.

This document also discusses the relatively new nature of professional doctorate programs, with the distinguishing factor being an emphasis on research application leading to preparation to function in advanced practice roles, as well as administrative, executive, public policy, and teaching roles. The AACN also stresses that the Nursing Doctorate (ND) degree, first offered at Case Western Reserve University in

1979, prepares individuals at the entry level for practice and is not a research-focused degree.

In 2002 AACN charged a task force to examine the current status of practice doctoral programs, assess the need for clinically focused doctoral programs, and clarify their purpose, core content, and core competencies. The resulting document stated that doctoral programs in nursing and other practice disciplines can emphasize either research or practice. It defined practice as "any form of nursing intervention that influences healthcare outcomes for individuals or populations including the direct care of individual patients, management of care for individuals and populations, administration of nursing and healthcare organizations, and the development and implementation of health policy. Preparation at the practice doctorate level includes advanced preparation in nursing, based on nursing science, and is at the highest level of nursing practice" (AACN 2004; http://www.aacn.nche.edu/DNP/pdf/DNP.pdf). The AACN Board of Directors accepted the report, recommended the establishment of Doctor of Nursing Practice (DNP) programs, and has since convened consensus meetings of doctoral faculty to forward this agenda for nursing education and nursing (AACN 2004). To date, 47 schools of nursing have accepted applicants to their DNP programs, and another 140 schools are considering or developing DNP curricula. In 2006, after a two-year consensus-building process, AACN member institutions voted to endorse *Essentials of Doctoral Education for Advanced Nursing Practice*. These Essentials are to be used in conjunction with competencies, content, and practical experiences needed for specific roles in specialty areas delineated by national specialty organizations for the development of curriculum and program evaluation. The eight essentials are:

1. Scientific underpinnings for practice;
2. Organizational and systems leadership for quality improvement and systems thinking;
3. Clinical scholarship and analytical methods for evidence-based practice;
4. Information systems/technology and patient care technology for the improvement and transformation of health care;
5. Healthcare policy for advocacy in health care;
6. Interprofessional collaboration for improving patient and population health outcomes;
7. Clinical prevention and population health for improving the nation's health; and
8. Advanced nursing practice. (AACN 2006, pp. 8–16; http://www.aacn.nche.edu/DNP/pdf/Essentials.pdf)

AACN has also created a new nursing role, Clinical Nurse Leader (CNL), to better meet client care needs within the healthcare delivery system (AACN 2007; http://www.aacn.nche.edu/Publications/WhitePapers/CNL2-07.pdf). The CNL is a leader or coordinator at the point of care to individuals, cohorts, or populations. The CNL:

- Designs, implements, and evaluates client care;
- Coordinates, delegates, and supervises the care provided by the healthcare team;
- Assumes accountability for client care outcomes; and
- Ensures the application of evidence-based practice.

The implementation of the role is expected to vary across settings.

Another interesting trend is that some community colleges that previously offered only associate degree education for nurses now offer baccalaureate degrees. This will expand the availability of baccalaureate nursing programs and increase the number of baccalaureate-prepared nurses nationwide. In response, AACN has released a *Position Statement on Baccalaureate Nursing Programs Offered by Community Colleges* (AACN 2005; http://www.aacn.nche.edu/Publications/positions/ccbsn.htm) which urges that these programs maintain the standards set by nursing's specialized accreditation agencies and emulate the liberal and scientific foundation of BSN programs offered in four-year colleges.

The **National League for Nursing** (NLN) is a national membership organization whose mission is to advance the quality of nursing education and ensure that it prepares the nursing workforce to meet the needs of diverse populations in an ever-changing healthcare environment. NLN sets standards to promote excellence and innovation in nursing education, professional growth and continuous quality improvement of faculty, research that informs and supports evidence-based teaching practices, and assessment and evaluation of educational outcomes and programs of nursing education. Unlike AACN, NLN supports all levels of educational preparation of the registered nurse, including associate degree and diploma programs.

To better serve the nursing community and address conflict of interest issues, NLN established the National League for Nursing Accreditation Commission (NLNAC) in 1997 as an independent subsidiary accountable to the NLN directly through the NLN Board of Governors. NLNAC provides accreditation of associate degree, diploma, baccalaureate, and graduate nursing programs.

In 2003 the NLN issued the position statement, *Innovation in Nursing Education: A Call to Reform* (www.nln.org/aboutnln/PositionStatements/innovation082203.pdf), which urged dramatic changes in both graduate and undergraduate nursing education to move from specific content and a clinical placement model of nursing education to an evidence-based curriculum that is flexible, responsive to student needs, collaborative, and integrates current technology. At about the same time, the NLN also convened a Think Tank on Perioperative Nursing in the Curriculum in conjunction with the Association of Perioperative Registered Nurses (AORN). The two organizations had identified a critical problem in nursing education: the removal of perioperative content from the curricula of most schools of nursing. The purpose of the think tank was to determine what knowledge, skills, and values associated with caring for perioperative patients and their families are appropriate to generalist education for the RN role (NLN 2004; http://www.nln.org/aboutnln/ProfOpportunities_11_09_04/innovation.htm).

The NLN Task Group on Nurse Educator Competencies identified eight competency domains for specialization as a nurse educator (NLN 2005a; http://www.nln.org/ProfDev/pdf/corecompetencies.pdf):

- Facilitate learning
- Facilitate learner development and socialization
- Use assessment and evaluation strategies
- Participate in curriculum design and evaluation of program outcomes
- Pursue continuous quality improvement in the nurse educator role
- Engage in scholarship, service, and leadership
- Function as a change agent and leader
- Engage in scholarship of teaching
- Function effectively within the educational environment and the academic community

Following this work, the NLN began offering the Nurse Educator certification exam in 2005.

In 2005 the NLN released a position statement entitled *Transforming Nursing Education,* a response to concern about the proliferation of mandates and proposals from various groups concerning nursing education. The statement acknowledges a complex and dynamic healthcare environment that demands new competencies of nurses. It identifies such drivers of transformation in nursing education as societal need, societal demand, and accountability for efficient and effective use of educational resources. However, NLN urges faculty "to base their curriculum designs, teaching/learning strategies, and evaluation methods on evidence-based standards and research rather than on politically driven pronouncements." The position statement further delineates ten recommendations in a call to action. One of those recommendations urges that "faculty identify themselves as advanced practice nurses since teaching is an advanced practice role that requires specialized knowledge and advanced education and since certification now exists as a way to recognize expertise in the role" (NLN 2005b; http://www.nln.org/aboutnln/positionstatements/transforming052005.pdf).

The **National Organization of Nurse Practitioner Faculty (NONPF)** has identified its charge to be the provision of leadership to promote quality nurse practitioner education at the national and international levels. Its research efforts identified five core competencies for nurse practitioner practice, originally published in 1990, revised in 1995 with the addition of another competency, and again revised in 2000 with the addition of a seventh competency. The core competencies document defines a patient as an individual, family, group, or community.

In 2002 NONPF published *Nurse Practitioner Primary Care Competencies In Specialty Areas: Adult, Family, Gerontological, Pediatric, and Women's Health.* The identified competencies for these nursing specialties reside in seven domains of practice:

1. Management of patient health/illness status
2. Nurse practitioner–patient relationship
3. Teaching–coaching function
4. Professional role
5. Managing and negotiating healthcare delivery systems
6. Monitoring and ensuring the quality of healthcare practice
7. Cultural competence (NONPF 2002b; http://www.nonpf.org/evalcriteria2002.pdf)

NONPF employed a collaborative process to identify the competencies. This involved a multi-organizational national panel that included an initial group who met to draft competencies and then forwarded the competencies to an external validation panel nominated by national organizations and composed of members who had not served on the first group. The competencies were reviewed for relevancy, specificity, and comprehensiveness. Following revision and consensus on the final document, NONPF distributed the competencies for endorsement by national nursing organizations linked to the project during the two development phases.

The original nurse practitioner primary care competencies were seen as setting the national standard for guiding program development in the five different primary care focus areas and providing the model for the future development of competencies for other specialty-focused nurse practitioner roles. Specialty, defined as the population focus, is not synonymous with specialty care, which may denote the clinical area of practice. The expectation is that these competencies will be used to guide curriculum development and revision nationally, as well as influence the credentialing and accrediting bodies.

In 2006 NONPF released a new edition of *Domains and Core Competencies of Nurse Practitioner Practice*, a significant revision of the 2002 version (NONPF 2006a; http://www.nonpf.com/NONPF2005/CoreCompsFINAL06.pdf). In response to feedback from nurse educators, this list of 75 competencies in seven domains reduced redundancy and facilitated measurement and evaluation. Only one domain name sustained a change—*cultural competence* was renamed *culturally sensitive care*. All nurse practitioners are expected to be able to demonstrate these core competencies at graduation. As with the earlier core competencies, specialty competencies are to build on this work.

NONPF has published other works on other competencies to help guide curriculum development, implementation, and evaluation, including the *Psychiatric-Mental Health Nurse Practitioner Competencies* (2003; http://www.nonpf.org/finalcomps03.pdf) and the *Acute Care Nurse Practitioner Competencies* (2004; http://www.nonpf.org/ACNPcompsfinal20041.pdf).

These entry-level competencies for graduates of master's or post-master's programs preparing the nurse practitioner for the specialty population emphasize the unique practice of the specialty and the needs of the population served; they are to be used in conjunction with the core competencies identified for all nurse practitioners. In addition, NONPF clearly states that this content should build on the graduate and advanced practice nursing core content identified in AACN's *Master's Essentials* to shape the nurse practitioner curricula.

NONPF's *Criteria for Evaluation of Nurse Practitioner Programs*, originally published in 1997 (http://www.nonpf.org/evalcriteria2002.pdf), provided a standard framework for the review of nurse practitioner educational programs, and it was designed to be used in conjunction with other criteria for accreditation of graduate programs and for specialty nurse practitioner programs. The criteria were used extensively but, as more nurse practitioner programs and specialties emerged, many questions arose about the meaning and intent of some of the criteria.

In 2001 the National Task Force on Quality Nurse Practitioner Education was convened to examine the relevance and currency of the criteria, and to revise and update these as necessary. NONPF and AACN circulated the updated criteria for endorsement by the nursing community. The 2002 edition of *Criteria for Evaluation of Nurse Practitioner Programs* included: forms designed to give nurse practitioner education programs a guide for developing their own tools to track data and perform their own program evaluation; a glossary of specialty courses and curricula and clinical and didactic learning experiences; standards of organization and administration; student admission, progression, grievance, and dismissal; curriculum requirements, including minimum clinical hours; resources, facilities, and services; faculty; and evaluation (NONPF 2002a; http://www.nonpf.org/evalcriteria2002.pdf).

In 2006 NONPF issued a position statement on the DNP. It states that the DNP is an important evolutionary step, but it does not support a finite deadline for transition of all nurse practitioner programs to the DNP (NONPF 2006b; http://www.nonpf.org/NONPF2005/PracticeDoctorateResourceCenter/CompetencyDraftFInalApril2006.pdf).

The **Association of Faculties of Pediatric Nurse Practitioners** (AFPNP), founded in 1972, is a national organization of nursing educators who teach in pediatric, family, and school nurse practitioner programs, and who work together on practice and educational issues. In 1978 the organization set goals and purposes following a national meeting about pediatric certification. AFPNP is the author of *Philosophy, Conceptual Model and Terminal Competencies for the Education of Pediatric Nurse Practitioners* (AFPNP 1996), used by pediatric nurse practitioner programs across the United States. It meets annually in conjunction with the National Association of Pediatric Nurse Associates and Practitioners (NAPNAP) yearly conference.

The **National Association of Clinical Nurse Specialists** (NACNS) was formed in 1995 to promote the unique practice of clinical nurse specialists (CNS) and to articulate practice, competencies, educational guidelines, and credentialing requirements for CNSs. The CNS is a registered nurse with graduate education (master's, post-master's, or doctorate) who is a clinical expert in the diagnosis and treatment of illness and the delivery of evidence-based nursing interventions (ANA 2004a). According to NACNS (2004, p. 12), CNSs have advanced nursing science knowledge with a specialty focus in a population (pediatric, geriatric, women's health), a type of problem (pain, wound management), a setting (critical care, operating room, emergency department), a type of care (rehabilitation, end-of-life), or a disease, pathology, or medical specialty (diabetes, oncology, psychiatry). NACNS further defines CNS practice as "targeted toward achieving quality, cost-effective outcomes through patient/client care, by influencing the practice of other nurses and nursing personnel, and by influencing the healthcare organization to support nursing practice" (p. 18).

The current CNS competencies are defined by the three spheres of influence: the patient or client, nurses and nursing practice, and the organization or system. Nursing process competencies are delineated in each sphere. A national task force composed of multiple specialty organizations with a significant investment in the CNS role is currently reviewing all CNS competencies for inclusion into a single set of role competencies. This work commenced in 2006 and is expected to be completed in 2008.

The NACNS recommends use of the AACN *Master's Essentials* for the nursing core content and the advanced practice nursing core, but recommends the following as additional content specific to CNS practice: theoretical foundations for CNS practice; theoretical and empirical knowledge of phenomena of concern that forms the basis for assessment, diagnosis, and treatment of illness and wellness within the CNS specialty; a theoretical and scientific base for the design and development of innovative nursing interventions and programs of care; clinical inquiry and critical thinking with advanced knowledge; selection, use, and evaluation of technology, products, and services; theories of teaching, mentoring, and coaching for use in all three spheres of activity; influencing change; systems thinking in regard to the organizational culture; leadership development for multidisciplinary collaboration; consultation theory; measurement; outcome evaluation methods; and evidence-based practice and research utilization (NACNS 2004, p. 43).

The **American College of Nurse-Midwives** (ACNM) has defined eight standards for the practice of midwifery (2003; http://www.midwife.org/display.cfm?id=485) and six core competencies for basic midwifery practice (2007; http://www.acnm.org/siteFiles/descriptive/Core_Competencies_6_07_3.pdf). These core competencies identify the knowledge, skills, and behaviors expected of a new practitioner, and this content must be offered in any education program seeking accreditation from the ACNM Division of Accreditation (DOA). Additionally, the ACNM has developed a scope of practice for the nurse-midwife specialty practice (ACNM 2005).

The **American Association of Nurse Anesthetists** (AANA) is the professional organization for certified registered nurse anesthetists (CRNAs). All nurse anesthesia programs are accredited by the Council on Accreditation of Nurse Anesthesia

Educational Programs (COA), which has served as the autonomous accrediting agency for nurse anesthesia programs since 1975. The Council is responsible for establishing standards and policies for nurse anesthesia programs, including: administrative policies and procedures; curriculum and instruction; the number and type of specialty anesthesia experiences required for graduation; faculty; and evaluation. The Council's scope of accreditation includes institutions and programs of nurse anesthesia at the master's, post-master's, and doctoral levels (AANA 2004).

Scope and Standards for Nurse Anesthesia Practice (2005; http://www.aana.com/uploadedFiles/Resources/Practice_Documents/scope_stds_nap07_2007.pdf) identifies 11 standards of practice, which include the nursing process and standards focused on documentation, infection control, patient rights, safety, and continuity of care. Competencies for the beginning nurse anesthetist include acquired knowledge and skills in patient safety, perianesthesia management, critical thinking, communication, and professionalism.

External Forces and Initiatives

Several notable initiatives outside the nursing profession have provided external influencing forces. The first Clinton administration's efforts for healthcare reform created quite a stir but failed to garner congressional support and funding. Having little success with these reform initiatives, President Clinton identified that the healthcare system was in need of change, and he constituted the Institute of Medicine's Committee on Quality of Health Care in America in 1998. He charged the committee to develop a strategy that would lead to substantial improvement in quality of health care over the next ten years. The work of this group and the subsequent reports produced have had tremendous influence on the current healthcare system and have resulted in significant efforts to change and improve the quality of the U.S. healthcare delivery system.

Institute of Medicine Reports

In 1999 the Institute of Medicine (IOM) released *To Err Is Human: Building a Safer Health System* (http://www.iom.edu/report.asp?id=5575). This landmark report has resulted in increased efforts to make our healthcare systems safer for patients and their families. The most often quoted statistics from this report are that medical errors are the eighth leading cause of death, with the deaths of between 44,000 to 98,000 Americans each year as a result of preventable medical errors, which are mostly system problems, not the fault of individual providers. The report estimated the annual cost of medical errors is $29 billion annually in lost income, disability, and healthcare costs.

The IOM's second report, *Crossing the Quality Chasm: A New Health System for the 21st Century* (2001; http://www.iom.edu/report.asp?id=5432), stated that "As medical science and technology have advanced at a rapid pace, the healthcare delivery system has floundered" (p. 2). "Between the health care we have and the care we could have lies not just a gap, but a chasm" (p. 1). This report found two major forces influencing the healthcare system: the constantly expanding knowledge base in health care and the increase in chronic care needs of the population.

The IOM suggested that the current healthcare system is inadequate and a fundamental change in the delivery of health care is necessary. The report gave ten rules for healthcare reform that included continuous health relationships, based on patient needs and values with the patient as a source of control, and stressed the need for knowledge sharing, free flow of information, evidence-based decision making, and safety. Additionally, it listed six key areas for improvement. The report suggested that health care needs to be:

- Safe – Avoiding injuries to patients from the care that is intended to help them;
- Effective – Providing services based on scientific knowledge to all who could benefit, and refraining from providing services to those not likely to benefit (avoiding underuse and overuse);
- Patient-centered – Providing care that is respectful of and responsive to individual patient preferences, needs, and values and ensuring that patient values guide all clinical decisions;
- Timely – Reducing waits and sometimes harmful delays for both those who receive and those who give care;
- Efficient – Avoiding waste, including waste of equipment, supplies, ideas, and energy; and
- Equitable – Providing care that does not vary in quality because of personal characteristics such as gender, ethnicity, geographic location, and socioeconomic status.

The IOM's third report, *Keeping Patients Safe: Transforming the Work Environment of Nurses* (2003b; http://www.iom.edu/report.asp?id=16173), called for an overhaul of the nursing work environment. It cited a substantial body of literature documenting the effects of fatigue on worker performance, including the effects of shift work and sustained operations on employee alertness. It suggested that actions are needed from the federal and state governments, as well as from coalitions of parties involved in shaping the work environments of nurses. The report's findings and recommendations addressed the related issues of management practices, workforce capability, work design, and organizational safety culture and recommended that nursing should:

1. Participate in decision making at all levels;
2. Promote evidence-based management practices;
3. Maximize the workforce capabilities of RNs and identify the need of RN staffing for each patient care unit per shift, recommending that staffing levels should increase as the number of patients increases and that nursing homes should have at least one RN on duty at all times;

4. Design work spaces to prevent and mitigate errors, limit nursing shifts to 12 hours in any 24-hour period and no more than 60 hours in a 7-day stretch; and

5. Create and sustain a culture of safety.

The IOM also published *Health Professions Education: A Bridge to Quality* (2003a; http://www.iom.edu/report.asp?id=5914), the conclusions of a health professions education summit in 2002 attended by over 150 leaders and experts from health professions education, regulation, policy, advocacy, quality, and industry. The summit focused on development of strategies for restructuring clinical education to be consistent with the principles of the twenty-first-century health system. The report said that physicians, nurses, pharmacists, and other allied health professionals are not being adequately prepared to provide the highest quality and safest medical care possible, and there is insufficient assessment of their ongoing proficiency. It also recommended that educators and accreditors, as well as licensing and certification organizations, should ensure that students and working professionals develop and maintain proficiency in five core areas: delivering patient-centered care, working as part of interdisciplinary teams, practicing evidence-based medicine, focusing on quality improvement, and using information technology.

Information Technology

Government-sponsored initiatives have been influential in driving technological advances in the capture, management, communication, dissemination, and storage of healthcare information. Efforts have focused on increasing the scope of electronic health records to encompass delivery and documentation of acute care, long-term care, and ambulatory care; provide access to evidence-based practice guidelines; and enhance the ability to measure and report outcomes. Access to electronic health records allows all providers of services to create better transitions to care and reframe care for patient populations. As this access evolves and expands, issues of privacy, confidentiality, and security must be considered and handled appropriately.

Another technological advance that has affected nurses and APRNs is the availability of computer-based examination technology. Prior to the 1990s, there were limited opportunities to acquire specialization credentials due to cost and security issues. Examinations to acquire specialty credentials were given in a paper-and-pencil format and were offered only once or twice a year at designated proctored testing sites. With the advent of computer-based examinations, a variety of certifications for professionals, including APRNs, has become more widely available. While NCSBN was able to develop NCLEX using computer-adaptive testing (each additional question in the examination is dependent upon a correct or incorrect response to the previous question), other certifiers with fewer financial resources have chosen to use computer-based testing (the examination is provided electronically to the test taker with all questions of a given form given to each test taker but in a random order).

Computerized testing both improved and provided new challenges to examination security breaches. It eliminates the need to have printed exams in circulation and the reliance on sometimes unreliable shippers. It ensures same-day turnaround, with no wait while used test booklets and score sheets are returned to the certifying agency for scoring. Computerized testing has also made testing more accessible, with the ability to be certified almost any time at any of 300 test centers around the country. It has eliminated the likelihood that nurses and APRNs can start employment before they have achieved a passing score on the necessary examination, and has thus made the certification and regulation of licensees more timely and valid. However, even as of 2008, there continues to be a lack of standardization and variable access, because not all APRN certifying exams are computerized.

Nursing Shortage Issues Drive Nursing's Agenda for the Future

The repeating cyclical shortages in the nursing workforce have affected many aspects of nursing and become an integral part of discussions about the adequacy of clinical education, numbers of bedside nurses, quality patient outcomes, an aging work force, and an aging nursing faculty. In an effort to remedy this shortage, Nursing's Agenda for the Future (NAF) was conceived and ultimately convened in September 2001. The 61 nursing organizations that attended included many specialty nursing organizations, reflecting the full spectrum of nursing interests and specialty practice. At the beginning of the summit, participants were challenged with this question: "You have been successful in addressing the problems nurses faced in 2001. How would you describe nursing in the year 2010?" The meeting's established work processes encouraged all to contribute, stimulated thoughtful discussions and consensus development, and created a synergy to craft a blueprint for nursing's agenda and action plans for the future. Unfortunately the final day's work sessions were abruptly halted by the events of September 11.

The vision statement developed at that summit remains applicable in today's environment:

> Nursing is *the* pivotal healthcare profession, highly valued for its specialized knowledge, skill, and caring in improving the health status of the public and ensuring safe, effective, quality care. The profession mirrors the diverse population it serves and provides leadership to create positive changes in health policy and delivery systems. Individuals choose nursing as a career, and remain in the profession, because of the opportunities for personal and professional growth, supportive work environments, and compensation commensurate with roles and responsibilities. (ANA 2002, p. 7; http://nursingworld.org/MainMenuCategories/HealthcareandPolicyIssues/Reports/AgendafortheFuture.aspx)

The participants also defined ten domains or areas of focus, as well as short-term targets that need to be addressed to bring about positive change for nursing and the healthcare system. The ten domains include:

1. Leadership and planning
2. Delivery systems
3. Legislation, regulation, and policy
4. Professional nursing culture
5. Recruitment and retention
6. Economic value
7. Work environment
8. Public relations and communication
9. Education
10. Diversity

The NAF Steering Committee, which formed the core of the effort, continued to meet after September 11 and led each of the domain groups and the many organizations in the development of action plans around each domain. Over time, efforts became more focused on those domains that were the drivers, such as the economic value of nurses. Many national nursing organizations, as well as state nurses associations, contributed financially to support the development of a model to describe and quantify the economic value of nurses. This work documented the difference in patient outcomes that cost hospitals money when a nursing unit is short-staffed by even one full-time registered nurse.

A Model for Defining Practice and Acceptable Competence

As new areas of specialty practice are recognized, and the accepted and traditional processes by which the profession manages itself are challenged, it seems important to provide a model that explains the role of various entities in defining the practice of the nursing profession. The members of the ANA Committee on Nursing Practice Standards and Guidelines have formulated a model to clarify the roles and relationships associated with regulation of nursing practice. The model recognizes the contributions of professional and specialty nursing organizations, educational institutions, credentialing and accrediting organizations, and regulatory agencies; clarifies the role of workplace policies and procedures; and confirms the individual nurse's ultimate responsibility and accountability for defining nursing practice. This model is relevant regardless of the degree or level of nursing being practiced along the continuum of care. New strategies and solutions for creating consensus about the level of legal or external regulation required can emerge from an examination and application of the model.

> ▍ *Definition of Nursing* – Nursing is the protection, promotion, and optimization of health and abilities, prevention of illness and injury, alleviation of suffering through the diagnosis and treatment of human response, and advocacy in the care of individuals, families, communities, and populations. (ANA 2004a, p. 7)

- *Definition of Scope of Practice* – The scope of practice statement describes the "who," "what," "where," "when," "why," and "how" of nursing practice. Each of these questions must be sufficiently answered to provide a complete picture of the practice and its boundaries and membership. The profession of nursing has one scope of practice that encompasses the full range of nursing practice. The depth and breadth in which individual registered nurses engage in the total scope of nursing practice is dependent upon education, experience, role, and the population served. (ANA 2004a, p. 1)
- *Definition of Standards* – Standards are authoritative statements by which the nursing profession describes the responsibilities for which its practitioners are accountable. Consequently, standards reflect the values and priorities of the profession. Standards provide direction for professional nursing practice and a framework for the evaluation of this practice. Written in measurable terms, standards also define the nursing profession's accountability to the public and the outcomes for which registered nurses are responsible. (ANA 2004a, p.1)

The nursing profession, including professional and nursing specialty organizations, must be responsible to its members and to the public it serves to define the scope of practice and standards of practice for nursing. This is foundational work that provides the basis for further description and refinement by other entities and is represented as the broadest level at the base of the pyramid in Figure 1-1.

The scope and standards of nursing practice and code of ethics serve as the foundation for legislation and regulatory policy-making that may be set in place to help assure the protection of the public's safety. This next level of the pyramid is represented by the Nurse Practice Acts and Rules and Regulations.

At the third level, scopes of practice, standards of practice, nurse practice acts, and rules and regulations guide development of institutional policies and procedures to create a more detailed representation of what constitutes safe, quality, and evidence-based nursing practice.

Finally, the registered nurse, using skills, knowledge, and professional judgment, ultimately determines what is appropriate nursing practice based on the scope of practice, standards of practice, nurse practice acts, legal regulations, and institutional policies and procedures. Although there may be opportunities for a more extensive practice, the registered nurse may elect a smaller subset. That level of self-determination will change over time, but always remains focused on the outcome being safe, quality, and evidence-based nursing practice.

Consider using a top-to-bottom approach to further understand the usability of the model. Imagine the registered nurse confronting a scope of practice problem or question unlike anything previously encountered. The registered nurse could seek guidance and clarification from the institutional policies and procedures. If the answer still proved elusive, the next step could involve examination of the applicable nurse practice act and regulatory language. This level of inquiry may involve formal

FIGURE 1-1 Model of Professional Nursing Practice Regulation:
Outcome = Safe, Quality, and Evidence-based Nursing Practice

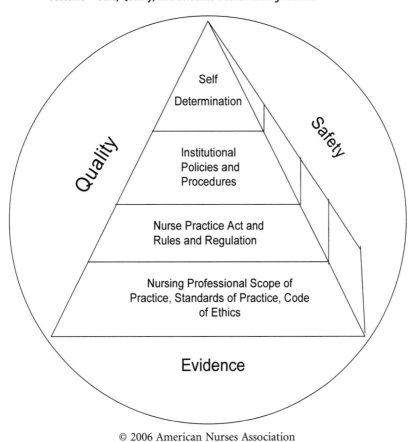

Self
Determination

Institutional
Policies and
Procedures

Nurse Practice Act and
Rules and Regulation

Nursing Professional Scope of
Practice, Standards of Practice, Code
of Ethics

Quality

Safety

Evidence

© 2006 American Nurses Association

consultation with the state board of nursing. Finally, review of the language embedded in the recognized professional scope and standards of practice and code of ethics may inform the decision about safe, quality, and evidence-based practice. Other stakeholders may also use the Model for Professional Nursing Practice Regulation in making practice decisions.

Summary

This chapter has highlighted some of the key issues, events, and decisions relevant to nursing and specialty nursing practice and regulation over the past two decades. The complexity of specialization and credentialing is demonstrated by the diverse perspectives of assorted organizations and interests. The profession is challenged to reach consensus about the future of credentialing and regulation that meets the needs of all nurses, including APRNs, and all specialties.

References

American Association of Colleges of Nursing (AACN). (1996.) *The essentials of master's education for advanced practice nursing.* http://www.aacn.nche.edu/Education/pdf/MasEssentials96.pdf.

American Association of Colleges of Nursing (AACN). (1998.) *The essentials of baccalaureate education for professional nursing practice.* http://www.aacn.nche.edu/Education/pdf/BaccEssentials98.pdf.

American Association of Colleges of Nursing (AACN). (2001.) *Indicators of quality in research-focused doctoral programs in nursing.* http://www.aacn.nche.edu/publications/positions/qualityindicators.htm.

American Association of Colleges of Nursing (AACN). (2002.) *Indicators of something or other in research-focused doctoral programs in nursing.*

American Association of Colleges of Nursing (AACN). (2004.) *Position statement on the practice doctorate in nursing.* http://www.aacn.nche.edu/DNP/pdf/DNP.pdf.

American Association of Colleges of Nursing (AACN). (2005.) *Position statement on baccalaureate nursing programs offered by community colleges.* http://www.aacn.nche.edu/Publications/positions/ccbsn.htm.

American Association of Colleges of Nursing (AACN). (2006.) *The essentials of doctoral education for advanced nursing practice.* http://www.aacn.nche.edu/DNP/pdf/Essentials.pdf.

American Association of Colleges of Nursing (AACN). (2007.) *White paper on the education and role of the clinical nurse leader.* http://www.aacn.nche.edu/Publications/WhitePapers/CNL2-07.pdf.

American Association of Nurse Anesthetists (AANA). (2004.) *Standards for accreditation of nurse anesthesia educational programs*

American Association of Nurse Anesthetists (AANA). (2005.) *Scope and standards for nurse anesthesia practice.* http://www.aana.com/uploadedFiles/Resources/Practice_Documents/scope_stds_nap07_2007.pdf

American Board of Nursing Specialties (ABNS). (2004.) *Accreditation standards.* http://www.nursingcertification.org/pdf/Standards-revised-10-04.pdf.

American College of Nurse Midwives (ACNM). (2003.) *Standards for the practice of midwifery.* http://www.midwife.org/display.cfm?id=485.

American College of Nurse Midwives (ACNM). (2005.) *Scope of practice of midwifery.* http://www.midwife.org/siteFiles/legislative/CNM-CM-CPM_chart_FINAL_March_07.pdf

American College of Nurse Midwives (ACNM). (2007.) *Core competencies for basic midwifery practice.* http://www.acnm.org/siteFiles/descriptive/Core_Competencies_6_07_3.pdf.

American Nurses Association (ANA). (2002.) *Nursing's agenda for the future.* http://nursingworld.org/MainMenuCategories/HealthcareandPolicyIssues/Reports/AgendafortheFuture.aspx

American Nurses Association (ANA). (2004a.) *Nursing: Scope and standards of practice.* Washington, DC: Nursesbooks.org.

American Nurses Association (ANA). (2004b.) *Scope and standards for nurse administrators.*(2nd ed). Washington, DC: Nursesbooks.org.

Association of Faculties of Pediatric Nurse Practitioners (AFPNP). (1996.) *Philosophy, conceptual model and terminal competencies for the education of pediatric nurse practitioners.* AFPNP.

Health Resources and Services Administration (HRSA). (2004.) *National sample survey of registered nurses.* http://bhpr.hrsa.gov/healthworkforce/reports/ rnpopulation/preliminaryfindings.htm

Institute of Medicine (IOM). (1999.) *To err is human: Building a safer health system.* http://www.iom.edu/report.asp?id=5575.

Institute of Medicine (IOM). (2001.) *Crossing the quality chasm: A new health system for the 21st century.* http://www.iom.edu/report.asp?id=5432.

Institute of Medicine (IOM). (2003a.) *Health professions education: A bridge to quality.* http://www.iom.edu/report.asp?id=5914.

Institute of Medicine (IOM). (2003b.) *Keeping patients safe: Transforming the work environment of nurses.* http://www.iom.edu/report.asp?id=16173.

National Association of Clinical Nurse Specialists (NACNS). (2004.) *Statement on clinical nurse specialist practice and education* (2nd ed.). Harrisburg, PA: NACNS.

National Commission for Certifying Agencies (NCCA). (2007.) *NCCA accreditation.* http://www.noca.org/Resources/NCCAAccreditation/tabid/82/Default.aspx.

National Council of State Boards of Nursing (NCSBN). (2007a.) *Home page.* https://www.ncsbn.org/index.htm.

National Council of State Boards of Nursing (NCSBN). (2007b.) *Nurse licensure compact administrators.* https://www.ncsbn.org/156.htm.

National League for Nursing (NLN). (2003.) *Innovation in nursing education: A call to reform.* www.nln.org/aboutnln/PositionStatements/innovation082203.pdf

National League for Nursing (NLN). (2004.) *Task group on innovation in nursing education.* http://www.nln.org/aboutnln/ProfOpportunities_11_09_04/ innovation.htm.

National League for Nursing (NLN). (2005a.) *Core competencies of nurse educators with task statements.* http://www.nln.org/ProfDev/pdf/corecompetencies.pdf.

National League for Nursing (NLN). (2005b.) *Transforming nursing education.* http://www.nln.org/aboutnln/positionstatements/transforming052005.pdf.

National Organization of Nurse Practitioner Faculties (NONPF). (2002a.) *Criteria for evaluation of nurse practitioner programs.* http://www.nonpf.org/ evalcriteria2002.pdf.

National Organization of Nurse Practitioner Faculties (NONPF). (2002b.) *Nurse practitioner primary care competencies in specialty areas: Adult, family, gerontological, pediatric and women's health.* http://www.nonpf.org/finalaug2002.pdf.

National Organization of Nurse Practitioner Faculties (NONPF). (2003.) *Psychiatric-mental health nurse practitioner competencies.* http://www.nonpf.org/finalcomps03.pdf.

National Organization of Nurse Practitioner Faculties (NONPF). (2004.) *Acute care nurse practitioner competencies.* http://www.nonpf.org/ACNPcompsfinal20041.pdf.

National Organization of Nurse Practitioner Faculties (NONPF). (2006a.) *Domains and core competencies of nurse practitioner practice.* http://www.nonpf.com/NONPF2005/CoreCompsFINAL06.pdf.

National Organization of Nurse Practitioner Faculties (NONPF). (2006b.) *Practice doctorate nurse practitioner entry-level competencies.* http://www.nonpf.org/NONPF2005/PracticeDoctorateResourceCenter/CompetencyDraftFInalApril2006.pdf

National Student Nurses Association (NSNA). (2007.) *Frequently asked questions.* http://www.nsna.org/membership/pdf/faq.pdf.

Chapter 2

Advanced Practice Nursing: Framework for Discussion of Issues, Goals, and Options

Margretta Madden Styles, EdD, RN, FAAN

Setting the Stage

Since the early developments in organizing specialties and setting standards for them, including the establishment of the American Board of Nursing Specialties in 1991, much attention has been focused on the advanced practice registered nursing (APRN) movement which has been gaining momentum. The education, certification, legal recognition, accreditation, practice, and political arenas have been buzzing with activities to accommodate this new growth within the body of nursing and health care. Unfortunately, these sectors haven't always worked fully in concert with one another. Thus, full empowerment has been compromised.

The four broad roles generally recognized as advanced practice registered nursing are nurse anesthetists, nurse midwives, clinical nurse specialists, and nurse practitioners. As a base for analyzing the situation, we can state in general terms the commonalities in advanced practice registered nursing. There are exceptions and dissenting opinions in each case.

- Advanced practice registered nurses are educated at the graduate level in institutions and programs accredited by state, regional, or national accrediting bodies.
- The knowledge and skills of advanced practice registered nurses are generally viewed as being along a continuum, in relation to the RN, thereby meriting expanded practice privileges and autonomy, as well as special reimbursement opportunities. Some visionaries might go beyond this concept to view advanced practice as the "new nursing" with entry level into nursing at the master's level.
- Advanced practice knowledge and skills are delineated and assessed according to national certification processes.
- Expanded practice privileges are legally recognized and in a number of states may be authorized through special licensure, sometimes called "a second license," which is in addition to the RN credential.

- Reimbursement through governmental programs and other entitlements is authorized by legislation at state and federal levels.
- Advanced practice registered nursing occurs across a range of healthcare settings and in a variety of organizational configurations, including collaborative and independent practice.

The APRN movement can realize its potential only if these functions are clear, coordinated, consistent, and mutually reinforcing. When one sector operates independent of the others, confusion, controversies, and inefficiencies result, creating bumps on the road to empowerment. For example:

- Universal positions, definitions, and classifications are lacking. At the one extreme are those who question whether advanced nursing practice in fact goes beyond the legal scope of the RN. On another front, there is widespread disagreement or uncertainty in operationalizing the concept of "specialties and subspecialties" in the advanced nursing practice arena.
- Domains, competencies, and standards for advanced practice nurse roles are variously defined within graduate curricula and certification, accreditation, and licensing bodies. In addition to the ensuing incoherence and redundancy in the system, nurses are subjected to inequities. Ideally there should be a smooth progression from graduation to certification to formal legal recognition to practice.

It is apparent that, although growth is dramatic, the very concept of the advanced practice registered nurse continues to evolve. On the one hand, this provides a splendid opportunity for the profession to develop its goals for the movement and the strategies for achieving those goals. On the other hand, it has created considerable upheaval for the movement.

The lack of consensus on the above issues reached a boiling point in 2004. The pot may have been stirred when the Texas Board of Nurse Examiners proposed to recognize nine "specialties" of nurse practitioners (NPs) and six "specialties" of clinical nurse specialists (CNSs). The Texas board may have made this unilateral decision out of frustration with the lack of leadership and direction in the profession as a whole. In addition, the action to "clean up ambiguity" may have been prompted by their interest in becoming part of the APRN Interstate Compact, which only one other state had joined at that time. Whatever the motivation, the move acted as a catalyst for a series of meetings and statements on the issues.

The American Nurses Association (ANA) and the American Association of Colleges of Nursing (AACN) co-hosted a conference of advanced practice nursing stakeholders in December 2004. Attending were representatives of educational institutions, professional associations, certifying bodies, regulatory agencies, and other interested parties. I was asked to open the meeting by laying out a framework within which discussions and decisions regarding advanced practice nursing issues could occur. The material presented in the rest of this chapter is essentially what I presented at that time, with limited additions. My intention is to update and refocus the issues and problems identified in the original publication on specialization in nursing, to identify the critical questions to be answered in developing a consensus around advanced nursing practice, and to propose criteria or goals for that consensus to meet. These questions will be posed in detail in Chapter 4.

Specifically, the objectives of the conference in December 2004 were:

- To discuss credentialing forms and interrelationships;
- To review existing and proposed divisions or specialties;
- To agree on assumptions and principles;
- To agree on a model for defining advanced practice divisions or specialties for regulatory purposes; and
- To draft a process for determining future divisions or specialties.

The following framework has been set within a context of specialization and credentialing. For decades credentialing, as broadly defined, has been my chosen medium for profession building and standard setting for nursing. Why? As will shortly be obvious, the stakeholders in the development of and standard-setting for advanced nursing practice—those represented in the meeting—are mostly credentialers (i.e., regulators) and they all play a critical role in the development of the profession and its education and practice standards.

Overview of Specialization and Credentialing

Credentialing Definitions and Characteristics

The term *credentialing* is used in both the national and international language of nursing. In the vocabulary of the International Council of Nurses (ICN), *regulation* is a common synonym for credentialing. It is applied in the majority of countries where standard setting is generally a governmental process, whereas the United States regulates through public–private partnerships. ICN uses the words *governmental* and *private or professional* as we use the terms *public* and *private* or *governmental* and *nongovernmental*. The term *credentialing* was popularized in nursing following the publication of ANA's *Study of Credentialing in Nursing: A New Approach* (ANA 1979). I was a central figure in both the ANA and ICN credentialing projects and developed the following conceptual base and definitions from those experiences:

- *Credential* – Documented evidence that an entity has met predetermined standards and requirements

▍*Credentialing* – An all-encompassing term applied to processes designating that an entity has met established standards set by an agent—governmental or non-governmental—acknowledged as qualified to carry out this responsibility

Some of the elements of credentialing and the ranges or options within them are as follows:

▍*Credentialed entity* – Individual, program, institution, or product
▍*Credentialing agent* – Governmental or non-governmental
▍*Credentialing jurisdiction* – Local, state, regional, or national
▍*Credentialing standards* – Minimal — safe, or above the minimum — superior; minimal standards are usually mandatory; superior standards are usually voluntary
▍*Credentialing purposes* – Public protection, title protection, quality improvement, or public recognition
▍*Credentialing forms* – Diploma- or degree-granting, licensure, registration, accreditation, approval, certification, endorsement, recognition, etc.

In general, the first five elements manifest in credentialing forms relate to nursing education and practice in the manner (there are exceptions) summarized in the table in Appendix A.

Complementarities among Credentialing Forms and Agents

This last form of credentialing listed—recognition by one credentialing agent of the credentials of another—is an important piece of the framework for addressing advanced nursing practice issues. In order to develop a stable, consistent, efficient, fair system for setting and implementing APRN standards, the potential and actual complementarities among the credentialing parties must be acknowledged:

Degree-granting institutions should recognize:

▍ Requirements for their graduates to qualify for certification and licensure (legal recognition) and
▍ Standards of accrediting agencies.

Regulatory/ Licensing authorities should recognize:

▍ National accreditation of schools for approving educational programs;
▍ Certification of advanced practice nurses for qualification for APRN licensure; and
▍ Accreditation of certifying bodies for assurance of the quality and reliability of their methods.

Certifying bodies should recognize:

▌ Accreditation of schools and programs to determine eligibility of graduates for certification and
▌ Guidelines of (regulatory) licensing bodies with respect to scope of practice and related competencies.

Accreditation and approval bodies for schools and programs preparing APRNs should recognize:

▌ Requirements of (state-legislated) licensing authorities and
▌ Requirements of certifying bodies.

True acknowledgment of these roles and complementarities would be reflected in procedures and requirements on the part of all "credentialing bodies" that are consistent in scope and quality, reliable in outcome, and comprehensive but not redundant.

Respective Roles and Mutual Recognition: Diagrams of Credentialing

Mutual Support and Recognition

This first diagram, Figure 2-1, illustrates how various forms of credentialing support one another in setting and implementing standards for advanced practice nursing.

▌ State (regulatory) licensing authorities are generally involved when a legal title (APRN) is granted and legal practice privileges are extended.
▌ National certifying bodies are engaged in identifying the knowledge and skill base for the area of practice, checking educational and experiential backgrounds, measuring competencies, and certifying that applicants are qualified.
▌ Certifying agencies are scrutinized by national accreditors or certifiers, just as schools of nursing are evaluated by national accreditors.

FIGURE 2-1 Mutual Support and Recognition

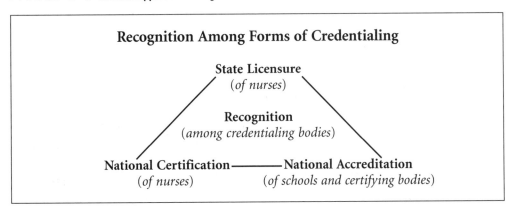

Recognition Among Forms of Credentialing

State Licensure
(of nurses)

Recognition
(among credentialing bodies)

National Certification———National Accreditation
(of nurses)   (of schools and certifying bodies)

FIGURE 2-2 Mutual Reinforcement

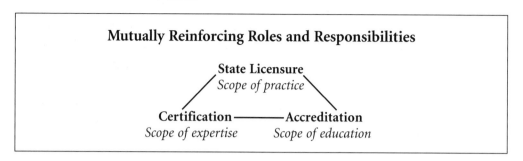

Through the process of recognition, all parties agree on requirements and methods and accept the appropriate role of counterparts or partners in credentialing advanced practice nurses. In effect, they are cross-referencing one another to create a seamless, reliable, comprehensive, non-duplicative process.

Figure 2-2 presents a concept of the core area of responsibility for each of the three credentialing authorities pictured above. State licensure must recognize a defined *scope of practice* to which licensees are entitled. Certification must reflect the *scope of expertise* (competence) required for that practice. Accreditation must ensure that the *scope of education* leads to the expertise required for the practice.

Figure 2-3 represents the array of functions that hold the system together. The agents, with their respective and complementary roles and responsibilities, must establish permanent, formal, and comprehensive mechanisms for communicating with one another. In these mechanisms cooperation, collaboration, and common agreements must be paramount. Means must be incorporated to confirm that each agent continues to meet expectations.

Powers of Credentialing

How does all of this translate into profession building?

In a June 2005 guest editorial in *International Nursing Review,* entitled "Regulation and Profession-Building: A Personal Perspective," published by the ICN, I explained the connection between the criteria for professions and the powers of credentialing:

FIGURE 2-3 Complementary Functions of Credentialing

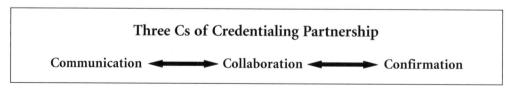

Only recently have I stepped back from operations to develop an enlarged vision of the critical role of regulation in profession-building. I have come to use the term *profession-building* in describing the struggle nursing has been engaged in since its origins to achieve the attributes and recognition of a true profession. Those attributes are generally accepted to be: (a) university (higher) education, (b) a distinct service or practice and discipline, (c) a research-based body of knowledge, (d) autonomy (self-governance) and accountability, (e) a code of ethics, and (f) an association to organize, serve, and speak for the members and the public welfare.

In search of the big picture as to achieving professional status, the question I asked myself is, "What is the relationship of those criteria to credentialing or regulation?" As one approaches, considers, and weighs the following *powers of credentialing* (referred to as regulation because of the international audience):

1. Regulation confers identity and continuity and universality upon our profession; it is a tie that binds us together.
2. Regulation is the major vehicle ensuring our accountability to the public.
3. Regulation defines our scope of practice and sets standards and measures of competency.
4. Regulation, through the use of explicit standards and processes, facilitates comparability and mobility among national and international jurisdictions.
5. Regulation authorizes us to use particular titles and present ourselves as such to the public.
6. Regulation removes our right to use particular titles and designations and our right to practice should we be found incompetent or unethical.
7. Regulation defines our body of knowledge by prescribing curricular content for schools and assessing the competence of graduates through testing and other means.
8. Regulation determines our degree of autonomy through granting or withholding various practice privileges to nurses.
9. Regulation establishes the minimum education requirement for those privileged to hold the title and to practice nursing.
10. Regulation explicitly or implicitly distinguishes between technical and professional occupations and significantly registers our progress as a profession, or lack thereof.
11. Many of the above powers, in combination, strongly influence the economic base of the profession.

(Styles 2005, pp. 81–82)

Combine the direct and indirect impact of the above forces and it becomes obvious that credentialing plays a major part in framing and buttressing the house of nursing.

A Global Perspective

In order to view our progress in advanced practice nursing within the context of our global profession, we should refer to the ICN and its International Advanced Practice Nursing Network. ICN has recognized regulation (credentialing) of nursing practice as one of its program pillars for several decades. The very recent establishment of such a network is recognition of the vital nature of the advanced practice movement as it reaches out around the world. We are not alone in struggling to bring order to the development.

ICN is rapidly producing publications to address circumstances confronting many of the 129 member nations. Documents have been published or are in process. The following excerpt is taken from *The Scope of Practice, Standards, and Competencies of the Advanced Practice Nurse* (ICN 2005, pp. 13–14):

Definition:

A Nurse Practitioner/Advanced Practice Registered Nurse is a registered nurse who has acquired the expert knowledge base, complex decision-making skills, and clinical competencies for expanded practice, the characteristics of which are shaped by the context and/or country in which s/he is credentialed to practice. A Master's degree is recommended for entry level.

Characteristics:

1. Educational Preparation
   - Educational preparation at advanced level
   - Formal recognition of educational programs preparing nurse practitioners/ advanced nursing practice roles accredited or approved
   - Formal system of credentialing, such as licensure, registration, certification, and credentialing
2. Nature of Practice
   - Integrates research, education, practice, and management
   - High degree of professional autonomy and independent practice
   - Case management/own caseload
   - Advanced health assessment skills, decision-making skills, and diagnostic reasoning skills
   - Recognized advanced clinical competencies
   - Provision of consultant services to health providers
   - Plans, implements, and evaluates programs
   - Recognized first point of contact for clients
3. Regulatory Mechanisms (country-specific regulations underpin NP/APRN practice)
   - Right to diagnose
   - Authority to prescribe medication
   - Authority to prescribe treatment

- Authority to refer clients to other professionals
- Authority to admit patients to hospital
- Legislation to confer and protect the title *Nurse Practitioner/Advanced Nurse*
- Legislation or some other form of regulatory mechanism specific to advanced practice nurses

The ICN standards do not include areas of focus or content; that is, they do not deal with specialty issues but consider advanced practice registered nursing as a role or core. Neither do they reference the four general categories of nurse anesthetists, nurse midwives, clinical nurse specialists, and nurse practitioners, as is true in the United States. Their purpose is to provide general guidelines for nations to adapt to their own needs. It seems wise to consider the basic framework, the fundamental characteristics advanced by our international colleagues, as we develop and refine the advanced practice registered nurse system for the United States, lest we weaken our ties to the global profession.

Summary of the Issues

The above sources and a cursory data analysis point to a number of definitional and credentialing issues that must be resolved if the advanced practice registered nurse movement is to progress toward professional empowerment. The issues are organized below in five general categories:

- *Definitional issues* – Debates range from definitions of advanced registered nurse practice to delineation of roles, specialties, and subspecialties within APRN practice. At present there is no defining concept or model to which all agree or conform; the very words *broad* and *narrow* have no common meaning.
- *Scope of practice issues* – There are majority and minority opinions as to whether the APRN scope of practice and privileges extend beyond those of the RN.
- *Issues related to educational standards* – There are majority and minority opinions as to graduate degree requirements for APRNs, with the vast majority favoring the master's or higher degree. Some schools do not seem inclined to follow specific curriculum guidelines for certification and licensure.
- *Credentialing issues* – The roles and responsibilities of, and the relationships among, credentialing (licensing, certification, and accreditation) bodies are in question.
- *Transitional issues* – Should we build on the base we have or start anew? As we make changes to the existing system, how shall we facilitate the transition for individuals and institutions?

Can we reach accord in the face of such controversies and uncertainties? We shall see.

References

American Nurses Association (ANA). (1979.) *The study of credentialing in nursing: A new approach.* Kansas City, MO: ANA.

International Council of Nurses (ICN). (2005.) *The scope of practice, standards, and competencies of the advanced practice nurse.*

Styles, M. (2005.) Regulation and profession-building: A personal perspective. *International Nursing Review,* 52(2), 81–82.

Chapter 3

Nursing Credentialing Now: Established and Emerging Specialties

Mary Jean Schumann, RN, MSN, MBA, CPNP

Advanced practice registered nurses (APRNs) today number over 240,000, according to the Nursing 2004 National Sample Survey (HRSA 2004; http://bhpr.hrsa.gov/healthworkforce/reports/rnpopulation/preliminaryfindings.htm). In 2007 APRNs are accepted as competent and qualified clinicians by millions of consumers who seek their care and often prefer it. Many physician colleagues consider APRNs a partial solution to the growing service needs of primary care, chronic care, underserved areas of the country, a dramatically aging population, an obstetric population whose specialists are overwhelmed by exorbitant malpractice insurance rates, and a variety of healthcare system woes.

Challenges to the Profession

APRNs have a malpractice claim rate that is less than 2%, many times less than their physician counterparts. The 2005 National Practitioner Data Bank Annual Report (http://www.npdb-hipdb.hrsa.gov/pubs/stats/2005_NPDB_Annual_Report.pdf) shows that physicians account for about 80% of health professional malpractice claims, and dentists account for another 13%. All other healthcare professionals, including nurses, account for only 8% of claims payments. Of that 8%, less than 2 out of 100 claims implicate APRNs, with nurse anesthetists responsible for 20% and nurse midwives responsible for 9% of all claims payments. Both past and recent research studies show that care provided by APRNs is every bit as high in quality as that of their physician colleagues (Mundinger et al. 2000; Mundinger & Kane 2000; Pinkerton & Bush 2000; Lenz et al. 2004; Lambing et al. 2004; Laurant et al. 2005; Sciamanna et al. 2006; Seale, Anderson, & Kinnersley 2006).

So what is causing the stress and the conflict in APRN practice?

APRNs have become much more visible to other health professionals with their increasing numbers and their insistence on taking their place in the world of healthcare reimbursement. This effort to capture third party reimbursement through entitlements such as Medicare, Medicaid, and commercial health insurers has caused physician groups and others to realize that significant revenue could go elsewhere.

The initiative to grant APRNs prescriptive privileges has likewise brought them unwanted attention. In the 1980s, nurse practitioners (NPs) began to seek support state by state for nurse practice acts and other legislative action on prescriptive authority. Eventually, state boards of nursing were obliged to acknowledge these movements and take some responsibility for the regulation of APRNs via their accountability to state nurse practice acts.

Even then, the increasing visibility of APRNs might have remained a non-issue, but eventually individual nurse practitioners were drawn into litigation. This raised questions such as whether they were appropriately prepared to provide such services, and what constituted the relevant education, the appropriate qualifications to sit for advanced certification, and the sufficient screening of such applicants. These questions led to the concern expressed at the national level by The National Council of State Boards of Nursing regarding whether certifying bodies provided psychometrically sound and legally defensible exams that adequately determined the safe practice of NPs.

Education and Certification

Dr. Styles's first edition of her book in 1989 was followed by several years of vigorous debate regarding sufficiency of education and the demonstration of minimum competence via examination and education, particularly focused on nurse practitioners. There were still a variety of mechanisms by which NPs could become educated, though that was changing. While master's level education had come to be a requirement for pediatric nurse practitioner (PNP) certification, other APRNs were not required to obtain master's degrees in their specialty and were not likely to be master's prepared. Candidates had been allowed to sit for certification exams for which they had not received the corresponding advanced education—for example, family, adult, or pediatric. Concerns emerged about the rigor of different certification examinations, and many questions were raised about discrepancies in educational programs, even at the master's level, with respect to numbers of clinical hours required and didactic content such as pharmacology, advanced physical assessment, and pathophysiology.

Not all advanced practice nursing roles were challenged in the mid-1990s to the same extent. Nurse anesthetists were presumed to be consistently educated in master's level programs. They were perceived to "work differently" and so were not an object of the challenges. Nurse midwives were not all educated within master's programs; this caused some consternation and enough pressure to force nurse midwives to adopt this minimum requirement by 2005. Clinical nurse specialists were also not challenged by boards of nursing, because they were assumed to be educated in master's programs and because they were far less likely to seek prescriptive privileges or obtain third party reimbursement. Their situation was also perceived to be more complex and therefore to be "saved for later."

Nurse practitioner regulatory issues took several years and many meetings and discussions to resolve. Finally, in 1997 it appeared that they had been solved through tightening of educational criteria for NP programs, stipulations that educational programs for each role would require master's degrees by a certain date, and agreement among the four advanced practice certifying bodies and NCSBN that each body certifying NPs would guarantee the soundness of their exam processes by seeking and achieving accreditation through the National Commission on Certifying Agencies (NCCA).

APRN Specialization

During the two decades since the first printing of Dr. Styles's book, many new specialties have surfaced, and more and more of them have advanced practice requirements and curricula. What had seemed a relatively clear-cut set of roles and educational options in the mid-1990s became complex in the eyes of nursing regulators in 2002. By then, a nurse who wanted to pursue a master's degree could become an NP or a CNS in specialties such as oncology, palliative care, or pain management. Regulators debated whether these were specialties or subspecialties, and what general advanced practice knowledge each graduate of these programs had obtained in addition to the unique knowledge of their specialty.

Graduates, instead of staying in the locale where they were educated and presumably accepted into the local practice community, were electing to move to other states where consumers, physicians, and, more importantly, boards of nursing were not familiar with their particular skill sets. Boards of nursing worried that graduates of such specialized programs who subsequently were unable to get a job as, for example, a palliative care NP or a pain management NP would then decide to seek employment as an adult or family NP and would not be qualified to practice as such.

Consequently, NCSBN, via its annual conference with state regulatory bodies, took a position in August 2002 to limit the proliferation of future exams and specialties. Specialty organizations and other professional organizations such as ANA protested this action, expressing serious concern that it would stifle the ability of the profession to adapt to new roles and specialties as population needs changed.

In 2004 the Texas Board of Nurse Examiners (TBNE) took the position that it would recognize only certain categories of nurse practitioners, namely adult, family, gerontology, pediatric, women's health, adult-acute care, psychiatric/mental health, and neonatal. Several long-established and widely acknowledged specialties for the CNS role were not included for recognition by the 2004 TBNE. Consequently, CNS programs for those specialties would close because those graduates would not be able to practice in Texas as CNSs. This position and the accompanying supportive rules were additional incentive for the larger nursing community to question the wisdom of letting a single state board of nursing set such precedents. National nursing organizations, such as ANA and AACN, urged that Texas delay adoption of these rules until the larger nursing community could address the issues that appeared to have prompted their actions. Despite this, TBNE continued to move forward.

However, in 2006 the Texas Sunset Advisory Commission made recommendations regarding TBNE's role. These included (TSAC 2006, pp.1–2; http://www.sunset.state.tx.us/80threports/final80th/79.pdf):

▌ Limiting the board's role to approving nursing education programs leading to initial licensure;
▌ Clarifying the board's authority to approve education programs already approved by other boards of nursing;
▌ Clarifying that nursing programs, once accredited by an agency recognized by the U.S. Department of Education, are exempt from board approval; and
▌ Adopting the Advanced Practice Registered Nurse Multistate Compact.

While the sunset recommendations are not yet final, it would seem that some of the measures to limit APRN practice will not be enacted.

Concurrently, other proposals for addressing the larger issues around advanced practice and regulation emerged nationally. In June 2004, AACN called together a group of nursing organizations, mostly composed of its AACN Alliance for Nursing Accreditation, members who represented certification, accreditation, and education of advanced practice registered nurses. The focus of this one-day APRN Consensus Conference was to initiate an in-depth examination of issues related to APRN definitions of practice, specialization, subspecialization, and regulation. Based on recommendations generated in the June 2004 Consensus Conference, the Alliance formed a smaller work group made up of designees from 23 organizations with broad stakeholder representation of APRN certification, licensure, education accreditation, and practice interests. The charge to the work group was to produce a statement that addressed the issues from the conference, with the goal of envisioning a future model for APRNs.

This group, now known as the Advanced Practice Registered Nurse Consensus Work Group, continues to meet to resolve conceptual issues relative to a futuristic model of regulation.

In December 2004, ANA convened a group of national nursing stakeholders, including members of this same APRN work group (listed on pp. 49 and 50), to discuss TBNE's position, with a goal of trying to convince TBNE to reconsider. Dr. Styles delivered a charge to this larger stakeholder group at the meeting: to think about a future-oriented model that would create a coordinated approach to the education, certification, regulation, and practice of APRNs. (See Appendix B for Dr. Styles' presentation.)

One outcome of the December 2004 national APRN stakeholder meeting was agreement that any organization that was not already a part of the APRN Consensus Work Group but wanted to join could do so. Furthermore, it was agreed that this group would take on the issues of regulation via an expedited consensus process. Some additional organizations did join. (These groups are listed in Appendix B, p. 73.)

The APRN Consensus Work Group also called attention to the need to clarify role competencies and educational standards for the CNS role. Some participants observed that a lack of consistency or clarity added significant confusion for state boards of nursing, making it impossible for them to determine which CNS specialties or subspecialties to recognize. This confusion about role competencies and educational standards, not evident in the other three APRN roles, was jeopardizing the practice of the CNS. A process for the larger CNS community to clarify and gain consensus would satisfy the needs of boards of nursing and others. This process is nearing completion by the CNS community, facilitated by ANA and ABNS.

The Work Group anticipated presenting a future-oriented document on regulation for endorsement by the APRN stakeholder community at a 2006 meeting at ANA headquarters. However, in February, 2006, NCSBN distributed a draft paper to the APRN stakeholder community on its vision of the future of APRN regulation. An NCSBN-sponsored APRN advisory panel composed of members of various boards of nursing worked on this draft document, which represented significantly different thinking than that of the Work Group. Many national nursing organizations provided feedback in writing to the NCSBN Board of Directors. The ultimate impact of that vision document remains to be seen. As of this writing, joint dialogues continue between NCSBN and representatives of the Work Group, with the goal of a single document to address the various factors that are required for successful and competent APRN practice. ANA, again with AACN, hosted another national meeting of APRN stakeholders in April 2008 to reach consensus on such a document. This book was written in part to help inform that debate and the future endorsement of a model.

Other Issues

Multiple controversial issues have surfaced from the APRN Consensus Work Group representatives and the NCSBN representatives in these discussions, including:

- Psychometric soundness of exams;
- Legal defensibility of the processes for determining eligibility for certification;
- Pre-accreditation of new APRN educational programs;
- Adequacy of clinical hours;
- Examination of core role content;
- Testing of content beyond the core relative to the population being served;
- Criteria for what constitutes a population versus a specialty for purposes of regulation; and
- Single or second scope of practice leading to licensure for APRNs.

This frequent and continuing dialogue, as well as feedback from the larger stakeholder community and input from various organizations with significant interests reflect diverse opinions about the solutions. This is to be expected when seeking consensus on a future-oriented solution for regulation of APRNs that provides reasonable assurance of a competent provider and protects the health of the public.

Physicians and Scope of Practice

A simultaneous threat to the practice of APRNs and other professional healthcare providers came from the American Medical Association (AMA). In November 2005 AMA accepted a resolution (Texas Resolution 814) at its House of Delegates to create a Scope of Practice Partnership to determine whether allied health professionals truly fill healthcare voids in rural and other underserved areas, and to closely examine the education and training of allied health professionals, providing this information as a point of comparison for legislators. Essentially AMA is challenging every "non-physician" provider group that threatens the physician reimbursement base.

The medical community has long perceived that everything that a physician does in the course of practice should be considered to be within only a physician's scope of practice. Barbara Safriet states "Once medicine's scope of practice was thus comprehensively defined in law, almost any activity directed at 'health or sickness'— especially if done for compensation—was deemed to be the practice of medicine. Licensed physicians then had obtained what sociologist Eliot Freidoson has aptly characterized as 'the exclusive right to practice.'" Safriet goes on to point out, "Under this skewed regime, even the simplest of everyday healthcare functions fell within the definition of medical practice, so no one else could do them absent the supervision of, or delegation by, a licensed physician" (2002).

Over the last 50 years the evolving roles of APRNs have challenged that perspective, as have the roles of other health professionals, such as chiropractors, physical therapists, and psychologists. Early versions of these roles were often based on unmet need and increasing access to health care for citizens who were otherwise unserved or inadequately served. Physicians and organized medicine have periodically fought the overlaps of practice with other health professionals, once again claiming all of the territory for medicine.

Boards of nursing have been pulled into this fray as their colleagues on boards of medicine have challenged the scope of practice for APRNs. In 2005 the Federation of State Medical Boards (FSMB) issued a position paper (http://www.fsmb.org/pdf/2005_grpol_scope_of_practice.pdf) that proposes that the FSMB develop an informational guide on patient safety and quality-of-care issues that should be considered by healthcare regulatory boards and legislative bodies when making decisions about changes in scope of practice. It would also assist when dealing with proposals to bypass established regulatory standards in order to extend healthcare services to undeserved areas. This document was unopposed by NCSBN who represented nursing in the position paper's development. ANA and AANA testified against this position.

In early 2006 many national nursing specialty associations and other health-related professional associations, such as physical therapy, came together to create the Coalition on Patients' Rights (CPR), for the purpose of countering the American Medical Association's scope of practice initiative which would limit patients' choice of health practitioners. In the face of organized medicine's latest divisive efforts to limit these professionals' abilities to provide the care and services they are qualified to give, CPR was formed for the sake of patients, to ensure that the growing needs of the American health system can be met and that patients everywhere have access to quality healthcare providers of their choice (CPR 2006; http://www.patientsrightscoalition.org/about).

As of this writing, there are numerous challenges to the practice of the fullest scope of nursing. While the nursing community has expanded roles and adopted a system of education, accreditation, certification, and legal recognition to ensure the competence of those who practice at this fullest scope, others threaten to restrict clinical practice for substantial segments of the APRN community, ostensibly to protect the public welfare and ensure safe care. There is little or no evidence that nurses or other allied health professionals jeopardize the care of their patients under the current regulatory system.

In June 2007 the AMA House of Delegates resolved to ask state and federal agencies to investigate the alliances between retail clinics and pharmacy chains; they emphasized conflicts of interest, risks to patients' welfare, and professional liability. The retail clinics have opened in the last few years to provide appropriately qualified and certified nurse practitioners to deliver limited episodic care on evenings or weekends when most primary care providers are not available. Retail customers can visit them for diagnosis and treatment of sore throats, respiratory infections, and a limited number of other ailments. The AMA House also committed to working to develop guidelines for model legislation to regulate store-based health clinics and will continue to monitor their development.

A Sample of Organizational Views

A number of organizations have stated positions on the controversial issues relating to measurement of competence, educational criteria, and scope of practice for advanced practice specialties. The following excerpts summarize the current debate and proposals, the organizational opinion, and dogma.

American Nurses Association (ANA)

ANA's *Nursing's Social Policy Statement* (ANA 2003) spells out nursing's responsibility to the public welfare. According to the latest edition,

- *Specialization* involves focusing on a part of the whole field of professional nursing. The American Nurses Association and specialty nursing organizations delineate the components of professional nursing practice that are essential for any particular specialty. Registered nurses may seek certification in a variety of specialized areas of nursing practice.

  Advanced practice registered nurses (that is, nurse practitioners, certified registered nurse anesthetists, certified nurse-midwives, and clinical nurse specialists) practice from both *expanded* and *specialized* knowledge and skills.

- *Expansion* refers to the acquisition of new practice knowledge and skills, including the knowledge and skills that authorize role autonomy within areas of practice that may overlap traditional boundaries of medical practice.

- *Specialization* is concentrating or delimiting one's focus to part of the whole field of professional nursing (such as ambulatory care, pediatric, maternal-child, psychiatric, palliative care, or oncology nursing).

  Advanced practice is characterized by the integration and application of a broad range of theoretical and evidence-based knowledge that occurs as a part of graduate nursing education. Advanced practice registered nurses hold master's or doctoral degrees and are licensed, certified, and/or approved to practice in their roles. (p. 9)

Among the important changes in the current edition of *Nursing: Scope and Standards of Practice* (ANA 2004a) is its integration of advanced practice issues throughout its content. In this resource, the APRN is defined as follows:

> Advanced practice registered nurses are RNs who have acquired advanced specialized clinical knowledge and skills to provide health care. These nurses are expected to hold a master's or doctorate degree. They build on the practice of registered nurses by demonstrating a greater depth and breadth of knowledge, a greater synthesis of data, increased complexity of skills and interventions, and significant role autonomy. As within all nursing practice, the level of expertise of the advanced practice nurse increases as they journey from novice to expert. (Benner 1982)

The document also addresses scope of practice:

> The profession of nursing has one scope of practice that encompasses the full range of nursing practice. The depth and breadth in which individual registered nurses engage in the total scope of nursing practice is dependent upon education, experience, role, and the population served. (p. 14)

Finally, *Nursing: Scope and Standards of Practice* defines measurement criteria for each standard of practice and professional performance for both registered nurses and advanced practice registered nurses.

ANA shapes its perspectives on advanced practice at least in part on the advice of an internal structural unit of the ANA, the Congress on Nursing Practice and Economics (CNPE). CNPE is key to the recognition of nursing specialties, approval of the nursing specialty's scope of practice, and acknowledgement of the specialty's standards of practice. A second internal ANA group that influences advance practice perspectives is ANA's Committee on Nursing Practice Standards and Guidelines, a standing committee of CNPE, charged with review and recommendations of nursing specialty scope and standards and guidelines.

American Nurses Credentialing Center (ANCC)

ANCC's processes for determining eligibility (master's level education) for APRN certification and producing psychometrically sound and legally defensible exams are predicated on the scope and standards of practice for that specialty practice, building on ANA's work. ANCC provides certification in a broad range of roles, populations, and specialties: adult NP; family NP; pediatric NP and CNS; gerontology NP and CNS; acute care NP; adult, family, and pediatric psychiatric and mental health NP and CNS; community health CNS; home health CNS; and others. ANCC is accredited by both ABNS and NCCA in recognition of the validity of their measurement processes for testing.

American Board of Nursing Specialties (ABNS)

The ABNS, recognized by the NCSBN for accreditation purposes, accredits specialty nursing certification programs, including those for advanced practice nursing specialties. Formal recognition by NCSBN as an accreditor of these programs denotes a significantly higher standard of legal defensibility and psychometric soundness of those certification examinations. The standard for definition and scope of nursing specialty reads:

> The certification examination program is based on a distinct and well-defined field of nursing practice that subscribes to the overall purpose and functions of nursing. The nursing specialty is distinct from other nursing specialties and is national in scope. There is an identified need for the specialty and nurses who devote most of their practice to the specialty.
>
> The eligibility requirement for advanced practice nursing certification includes a minimum of a graduate degree in nursing or the appropriate equivalent, including content in the specified area of specialty practice. (ABNS 2004; http://www.nursingcertification.org/pdf/Standards-revised-10-04.pdf)

American Association of Colleges of Nursing (AACN)

AACN has provided the *Master's Essentials* for defining the appropriate core content for APRN education (1996; http://www.aacn.nche.edu/Education/pdf/MasEssentials96.pdf). For AACN, the master's curriculum is conceptualized as having three components:

- *Graduate nursing core* — Foundational curriculum content deemed essential for all students who pursue a master's degree in nursing regardless of specialty or functional focus
- *Advanced practice nursing core* — Essential content to provide direct patient or client services at an advanced level, advanced health assessment, pharmacology, and pathophysiology
- *Specialty curriculum content* — Clinical and didactic learning experiences identified and defined by the specialty nursing organization

The Commission on Collegiate Nursing Education and the National League for Nursing Accreditation Commission, as discussed in Chapter 1, both accredit graduate-level nursing education programs, specifically for nurse practitioners and clinical nurse specialists. In that role, accreditation bodies are expected to verify the presence of specific program content and outcomes. Neither accreditor provides for pre-approval of new nursing education programs before admission of students to that program. This has drawn criticism as it can leave students disadvantaged after graduation because they do not meet necessary eligibility requirements to sit for certification. Nurse Anesthesia and Nurse Midwifery programs do require pre-approval of the program before admitting students and do not face this criticism.

National Organization of Nurse Practitioner Faculties (NONPF)

The National Organization of Nurse Practitioner Faculties has worked over the last 12 years to build consensus on core competencies and minimum educational criteria for nurse practitioner practice among all NP certifiers and programs. The NONPF website provides links to the following NP competencies:

- Domains and Core Competencies (2006; http://www.nonpf.com/NONPF2005/CoreCompsFINAL06.pdf)
- Psychiatric-Mental Health Nurse Practitioner (2003; http://www.nonpf.org/finalcomps03.pdf)
- Acute Care Nurse Practitioner Competencies (2004; http://www.nonpf.org/ACNPcompsfinal20041.pdf)
- Nurse Practitioner Primary Care Competencies in Specialty Areas: adult, family, gerontological, pediatric, women's health, and psychiatric-mental health (2002 and 2003; http://www.nonpf.org/finalaug2002.pdf, http://www.nonpf.org/finalcomps03.pdf)

National Association of Clinical Nurse Specialists (NACNS)

NACNS brings these positions to the discussion of APRN practice:

- CNSs have always been educated at the master's level.
- CNSs practice autonomously under the authority granted by the registered nurse license.

- CNSs expand the depth and breadth of nursing practice within existing autonomous authority.
- Prescriptive authority may be a characteristic of some CNSs' individual practice, but it is not a defining characteristic of CNS practice, meaning that use of prescriptive authority for CNSs is optional.

Other APRN Population Issues

One of the dilemmas in determining a futuristic model for credentialing has been the sometimes seemingly insignificant differentiation between NP and CNS practice in certain specialty populations. In such cases, the roles of NP and CNS merge to appear as a blended role. In others there have been practical decisions to declare oneself as an NP rather than a CNS in order to attain prescriptive authority and third-party reimbursement.

One example of this dilemma surrounds the psychiatric-mental health APRN. Currently, these APRNs may be either an NP or CNS, and in a given state they may only be recognized in one or the other of those roles. The other question that arises around the scope of practice of the psychiatric NP is whether they can treat the full range of adult issues. Does the psychiatric APRN have education across the adult spectrum of illness, or is the education largely psychiatric-mental health?

APRNs in oncology have similar practice issues. The Oncology Nursing Certification Commission currently provides certification for both the oncology CNS and oncology NP for the Oncology Nursing Society. This certification commission states that oncology CNSs and oncology NPs share a substantial core of knowledge important to both roles. However, there are discernable differences in work responsibilities for the NP and CNS in oncology. In terms of scope of practice, the question arises again: Is the oncology NP educated to deal with a wide range of health problems of the adult or the pediatric population?

One other issue with regard to scope of practice in particular deals with how APRNs are educationally prepared along the wellness–illness continuum. Several programs and certifying bodies credential APRNs as acute care or primary NPs. However, there is a blurring of the line between acute and primary care when NPs move among settings. In some states NPs can move more easily to other settings. For example, an adult primary care NP may provide care in a long-term setting. This raises the concern about competency in the other setting. The ANCC, The Pediatric Nursing Certification Board, The American Academy of Nurse Practitioners, and the American Association of Critical Care Nurses all credential NPs that may find themselves with this dilemma.

National Council of State Boards of Nursing

The NCSBN states that broad preparation for APRNs should be considered the minimum preparation for entry into advanced practice nursing to satisfy legal regulations. NCSBN has been opposed to the proliferation of what they term subspecialty programs, because graduates of these programs expect to be licensed as APRNs and legal recognition of narrow scope is inappropriate.

Some educational programs may wish to emphasize subspecialties as an appropriate educational direction. However, from the viewpoint of licensure, it is important to continue to meet the criteria for certification and subsequent licensure in the broader category. Certifying bodies also provide examinations in areas other than those intended for licensure. These "value-added" certifications offer a means of documenting special competencies within a practice area of an existing license. This use of certification is separate from purposes of licensure. The definitions used by NCSBN (2007; https://www.ncsbn.org/index.htm) are:

▎ *Specialty.* A broad, population-based focus of study encompassing common problems of that group of patients and likely comorbidities, interventions, and responses to those problems; e.g., neonatal, child, women, adult, family, mental health, anesthesia, and midwifery. (These are *not* specific diseases or health problems or specific interventions.)
▎ *Subspecialty.* A focus of practice within a specialty assuring expert knowledge of a particular area of patient problem: cardiovascular disease, palliative care, oncology, substance abuse, orthopedics, critical care, etc.

The NCSBN expects the APRN to complete an accredited master's program of study in a specialty area, take a nationally recognized certification exam in that area, and practice in that specialty. NCSBN, in addition to the Interstate RN compact, has developed an APRN compact to allow for mobility of APRNs among states. However, a hallmark of the approach is a requirement that all APRNs receive a second license in addition to their RN license, which is highly controversial and is opposed by some in the APRN stakeholder community. The NCSBN also states that APRNs have an expanded scope of practice which includes the RN scope. The scope is defined as advanced assessment, diagnosis, prescribing, selecting, administering, and dispensing therapeutic measures, including over-the-counter, legend, and controlled substances within the role and specialty-appropriate education and certification.

NCSBN has identified its own set of APRN regulatory principles. These principles must be addressed by the ARPN stakeholder community as part of the process of gaining consensus about a future-oriented model for APRN regulation:

▎ Scope of education, certification, and practice are congruent.
▎ Role and title should reflect educational preparation and examination.
▎ APRN licensure is necessary because the scope of practice exceeds the RN scope.
▎ Boards must approve educational programs leading to licensure.
▎ APRNs must graduate from approved programs in the specialty.
▎ Licensing examinations must be acceptable to boards of nursing.
▎ Examinations leading to licensure must be legally defensible and psychometrically sound. Content validity must be based on a job analysis.
▎ All educational programs leading to licensure must be accredited.

- Each track in a dual-track program must have a minimum of 500 clinical hours.
- The APRN specialty must consist of a broad population-based course of study.
- Curricula should be standardized and based on nationally recognized core competencies.

Summary

The evolution of multiple advanced practice roles over the last 60 years has created a complex array of expectations for academic preparation, outcome competencies, skill sets, and methods for ascertaining and ensuring acceptably safe practice. Even the responsibility for who measures and declares APRNs safe has changed dramatically over that time.

In spite of this conglomeration of approaches, all organizations are in agreement regarding the importance of safe practice and the welfare of the consumer. NCSBN would say it is their sole purview to ensure the public welfare. Yet all certifying bodies, and indeed educational programs and professional associations, would contend that the responsibility is shared by each of them as well. The approaches have worked very well, as demonstrated by the data regarding malpractice claims and errors. Some would ask, "Why work to fix a system that is not broken?" Yet, there are many who are disadvantaged by the scenarios that have been provided. And while organized medicine would like to think otherwise, APRNs are one solution to any significant move forward by this country regarding health systems reform.

Fortunately, this widely accepted commitment to safe care by APRNs is creating the glue for dialogue that will lead to a future-oriented model. It is very likely that each stakeholder engaged in seeking a common model will need to acquiesce to some level of change or compromise in approaches. The challenge is for each of the stakeholders to persevere to reach consensus on the concepts and the practical implementation of such a model despite the diversity of views and approaches.

Diversity and dissension characterize today's regulatory and credentialing environment for nursing practice. We have two options: Let this patchwork of diverse positions perpetuate discontinuity, or reconcile and refine them to present a unified system of specialization, credentialing, and regulatory processes.

References

American Association of Colleges of Nursing (AACN). (1996.) *The essentials of master's education for advanced practice nursing.* http://www.aacn.nche.edu/Education/pdf/MasEssentials96.pdf.

American Board of Nursing Specialties (ABNS). (2004.) *Accreditation standards.* http://www.nursingcertification.org/pdf/Standards-revised-10-04.pdf.

American Nurses Association (ANA). (2003.) *Nursing's social policy statement* (2nd ed.). Washington, DC: Nursesbooks.org.

American Nurses Association (ANA). (2004a.) *Nursing: Scope and standards of practice.* Washington, DC: Nursesbooks.org.

Coalition for Patients' Rights (CPR). (2006.) *About us.* http://www.patientsrightscoalition.org/about.

Federation of State Medical Boards (FSMB). (2005.) *Assessing scopes of practice in health care delivery: Critical questions in assuring public access and safety.* http://www.fsmb.org/pdf/2005_grpol_scope_of_practice.pdf.

Health Resources and Services Administration (HRSA). (2004.) *National sample survey of registered nurses.* http://bhpr.hrsa.gov/healthworkforce/reports/rnpopulation/preliminaryfindings.htm

Lambing, A.Y., Adams, D.L., Fox, D.H., & Divine, G. (2004.) Nurse practitioners' and physicians' care activities and clinical outcomes with an inpatient geriatric population. *J Am Acad Nurse Pract, 16*(8), 343–352.

Laurant, M., Reeves, D., Hermens, R., Braspenning, J., Grol, R., & Sibbald, B. (2005.) Substitution of doctors by nurses in primary care. *Cochrane Database Syst Rev, 18*(2), CD001271.

Lenz, E.R., Mundinger, M.O., Kane, R.L., Hopkins, S.C., & Lin, S.X. (2004.) Primary care outcomes in patients treated by nurse practitioners or physicians: Two-year follow-up. *Med Care Res Rev, 61*(3), 332–351.

Mundinger, M.O., & Kane, R.L. (2000.) Health outcomes among patients treated by nurse practitioners or physicians. *JAMA, 283*(19), 2521–2524.

Mundinger, M.O., Kane, R.L., Lenz, E.R., Totten, A.M., Tsai, W.Y., Cleary, P.D., et al. (2000.) Primary care outcomes in patients treated by nurse practitioners or physicians: A randomized trial. *JAMA, 283*(1), 59–68.

National Council of State Boards of Nursing (NCSBN). 2007. *Some title of some source for at least the NCSBN definitions of specialties and sub-specialties.* https://www.ncsbn.org/index.htm

National Organization of Nurse Practitioner Faculties (NONPF). (2002.) *Nurse practitioner primary care competencies in specialty areas: Adult, family, gerontological, pediatric and women's health.* http://www.nonpf.org/finalaug2002.pdf.

National Organization of Nurse Practitioner Faculties (NONPF). (2003.) *Psychiatric-mental health nurse practitioner competencies.* http://www.nonpf.org/finalcomps03.pdf.

National Organization of Nurse Practitioner Faculties (NONPF). (2004.) *Acute care nurse practitioner competencies.* http://www.nonpf.org ACNPcompsfinal20041.pdf.

National Organization of Nurse Practitioner Faculties (NONPF). (2006.) *Domains and core competencies of nurse practitioner practice.* http://www.nonpf.com/NONPF2005/CoreCompsFINAL06.pdf.

National Practitioner Data Bank. (2005.) *Annual report.* http://www.npdb-hipdb.hrsa.gov/pubs/stats/2005_NPDB_Annual_Report.pdf

Pinkerton, J.A., & Bush, H.A. (2000.) Nurse practitioners and physicians: Patients' perceived health and satisfaction with care. *J Am Acad Nurse Pract, 12*(6), 211–217.

Safriet, B. (2002.) Closing the gap between "can" and "may" in health-care providers' scopes of practice: A primer for policymakers. *Yale Journal on Regulation, 19*(2), 301–334.

Sciamanna, C.N., Alvarez, K., Miller, J., Gary, T., & Bowen, M. (2006.) Attitudes toward nurse practitioner-led chronic disease management to improve outpatient quality of care. *Am J Med Qual, 21*(6), 375–381.

Seale, C., Anderson, E., & Kinnersley, P. (2006.) Treatment advice in primary care: A comparative study of nurse practitioners and general practitioners. *J Adv Nurs, 54*(5), 534–541.

Styles, M. (1989.) *On specialization in nursing: Toward a new empowerment.* Kansas City, MO: American Nurses Foundation.

Texas Sunset Advisory Commission (TSAC). (2006.) Texas board of nurse examiners. http://www.sunset.state.tx.us/80threports/final80th/79.pdf.

APRN Consensus Process Work Group:
Representatives of the Organizations at the Work Group Meetings

Jan Towers, American Academy of Nurse Practitioners Certification Program

Joan Stanley, American Association of Colleges of Nursing

Carol Hartigan, American Association of Critical Care Nurses Certification Corporation

Leo LeBel, American Association of Nurse Anesthetists

Bonnie Niebhur, American Board of Nursing Specialties

Peter Johnson and Elaine Germano, American College of Nurse-Midwives

Mary Jean Schumann, American Nurses Association

Mary Smolenski, American Nurses Credentialing Center

M.T. Meadows, American Organization of Nurse Executives

Edna Hamera and Sandra Talley, American Psychiatric Nurses Association

Elizabeth Hawkins-Walsh, Association of Faculties of Pediatric Nurse Practitioners

Jennifer Butlin, Commission on Collegiate Nursing Education

Laura Poe, APRN Compact Administrators

Betty Horton, Council on Accreditation of Nurse Anesthesia Educational Programs

Kelly Goudreau, National Association of Clinical Nurse Specialists

Fran Way, National Association of Nurse Practitioners in Women's Health, Council on Accreditation

Mimi Bennett, National Certification Corporation

Kathy Apple, National Council of State Boards of Nursing

Grace Newsome and Sharon Tanner, National League for Nursing Accrediting Commission

Kitty Werner and Ann O'Sullivan, National Organization of Nurse Practitioner
    Faculties
Cyndi Miller-Murphy, Oncology Nursing Certification Corporation
Janet Wyatt, Pediatric Nursing Certification Board
Carol Calianno, Wound, Ostomy and Continence Nursing Certification Board
Irene Sandvold, DHHS, HRSA, Division of Nursing (*observer*)

Chapter 4

Reaching Accord: Parties, Principles, and Processes

Margretta Madden Styles, EdD, RN, FAAN

What Does It Take?

Reaching accord depends upon the open commitment of all key stakeholders or parties to agree on underlying principles and to establish the structures and processes to put the principles into effect.

To promote favorable attitudes underlying "commitment," we might first consider the dictionary definition of stakeholder: "One who holds money for others and pays it to the winner." Is that what we are? If we choose to apply the term to ourselves, let us work to ensure that we are all winners. Should we, could we, will we make that our goal? We must.

A better definition of stakeholder (even the dictionary says that the above definition is the "old" definition) is ". . . people who will be affected by an endeavor and can influence it but who are not directly involved with doing the work or people who are (or might be) affected by any action taken by an organization or group" (Wikipedia, online).

Parties

Professional associations formulate broad definitions and standards for the profession. Within these general guidelines, the parties directly involved in the credentialing of specialists and advanced practice registered nurses have been previously identified as educational institutions, accrediting agencies, certifying bodies, and regulatory and licensing boards. In fact, these groups largely empower the specialty movements. Upon reaching accord about principles and processes, they must then convene some form of council to carry out and maintain their agreements. For purposes of stability and maintaining momentum, this collective must be formal, permanent, and for this purpose only.

Principles

Let us begin with the principles that would underlie a prototypic advanced practice nursing model. Here is a draft list for review and modification. A model system should observe the following principles:

- ▌ Relevance and validity – The system is relevant to healthcare and work setting needs, and to the career paths of nurses.
- ▌ Purposefulness – Parties have an overt purpose and adhere to that purpose.
- ▌ Efficacy – Parties fulfill that purpose, producing intended results.
- ▌ Efficiency – Parties are able to fulfill purposes with appropriate effort, cost, resources, and minimum duplication.
- ▌ Consistency and reliability – Parties use consistent procedures and produce reliable results.
- ▌ Collaboration – Parties work in a network of partner organizations in setting and enforcing standards for practice.
- ▌ Accountability – Partners establish mechanisms for ensuring accountability to one another for fulfilling their purposes.
- ▌ Justice – Parties incorporate procedures for ensuring justice for all credentialed entities and applicants.
- ▌ Clarity – Systems are clear and comprehensible to nurses, consumers, and the public.
- ▌ Adaptability – Strategic planning and cooperative efforts anticipate, promote, and facilitate growth and change.
- ▌ Universality – To a feasible and appropriate extent, parties adhere to universal standards and definitions within the worldwide profession.

How many of the above principles would our U.S. "model" of nursing specialization and credentialing satisfy today?

Questions

Let us keep these principles in mind as we examine options for resolving these issues. First, we must translate the issues into specific questions, which the profession is challenged to answer.

Definitional Issues

Debates range from definitions of advanced practice to definitions or delineation of roles, specialties, and subspecialties in advanced practice registered nursing. At present there is no defining concept or model to which all agree or conform; the very words *broad* and *narrow* have no common meaning.

- Is there one core or base for advanced practice nursing along the lines of the ICN guidelines (e.g., definition and characteristics) and other sources? Are there four cores based on the four roles identified in the United States: nurse anesthetists, nurse midwives, clinical nurse specialists, and nurse practitioners? Or is there no core?
- Is there a conceptual framework for distinguishing core from specialty, broad from narrow, specialty from subspecialty? Are core, specialty core, and subspecialty additive or independent and self-contained; that is, are specialties built on the core, or do they stand alone?

Scope of Practice Issues

There are two articulated opinions regarding the scope of practice of registered nurses. One is that the APRN's scope of practice and privileges extend beyond those of the RN, as is implied in the term *advanced practice*. The other, and most often cited, position is that there is one scope of practice for all registered nurses that includes APRN practice, which contracts and expands according to the ongoing education, certification, and experience of the RN.

Issues of Educational Standards

There are majority and minority opinions as to graduate degree requirements for APRNs. The AACN *Masters Essentials* (1996; http://www.aacn.nche.edu/Education/pdf/MasEssentials96.pdf) and the NONPF *Criteria* (2002; http://www.nonpf.org/evalcriteria2002.pdf) very clearly direct educational programs to provide certain content, clinical hours, and experiences for their graduates to be qualified to take a certification examination upon degree completion. However, if a graduate program does not lead to national certification in the specialty, has it been made clear to the student that certification is not yet an option for this specialty?

Credentialing Issues

The roles, responsibilities, and relationships of credentialing (licensing, certification, and accreditation) bodies are in question.

1. Following the general pattern for health professionals, should state boards provide APRN licenses at the role level only, e.g., distinct cores for the nurse anesthetist, for the nurse midwife, for the clinical nurse specialist, and for the nurse practitioner?
2. Should state boards license at the level of "broad" advanced practice specialties, such as adult, pediatric, or geriatric? If so, does this limit the scope of practice to that broad area? By what concept and process are these broad areas determined? For example, if they are "population-based," how is *population* defined? Or should they be age based? Should they be made uniform for all states? By what process?

3. Should state boards recognize advanced practice registered nurses who practice in narrow specialty areas, e.g., skills, treatments, illnesses? Should secondary certification be required for narrow specialty areas?
4. How can the profession best be assured that certifying bodies are reliably and validly assessing competencies of candidates for licensure for core or broad areas of advanced practice nursing at entry and on an ongoing basis?
5. What content should certifying bodies measure? Is it APRN content, role content, population content, or specialty content? Should this all be in one exam, or should examinations be modular?
6. Should examinations, and examinations alone, be the means for measuring competencies? Can portfolios or other measures be adopted?

Transitional Issues

If we decide to make changes, should we build on the base we have or start anew? As we make changes to the existing system, how shall we facilitate the transition for individuals and institutions?

1. Should the building of a model for the future rest on ethical, political, or logistic grounds? What are the priorities?
2. What adaptation processes would facilitate change in the healthcare system to accommodate new models of nursing specialties?
3. What mechanisms would facilitate the transition of currently credentialed nurses into new specialization models?

The Possibilities

Having put forth the principles, issues, and questions as a framework for decision making, it is now time to hone in on the possibilities. For this purpose, the term *models* will be useful. Models include the specialization schema (concepts, categories, and divisions) and the related credentialing mechanisms by which such schema are implemented.

Models

There are two basic models: generic and specialized. What we have today could perhaps best be described as a historical model, shaped by the past, as circumstances and opportunities presented themselves. There has been little, if any, centralized policy-making and no overriding rationale, no grand plan to which the profession can be said to have agreed. In fact, among the principal parties there is no common understanding of the terms *generic* and *specialty*.

In simplest terms, the very title *advanced practice registered nurse* carries the connotation to nurses, consumers, and other health professionals of beyond the norm in education, competencies, and practice. If the profession does not intend to convey that message, perhaps another title is in order. And if the profession doesn't intend to recognize those nurses who are especially qualified, one might wonder why, particularly in view of the public's demand to know about those from whom they are receiving services.

Gradations of Generic Models

A purely generic model would title and license one category, e.g., advanced practice registered nurse, just as we have historically had the title and license of registered nurse. To this date the advanced practice nursing credential has been added to the RN. It would be possible, of course, to admit candidates to advanced nursing practice and licensure through programs preparing specifically for this purpose. Such persons would not be RNs and would not be titled APRNs. Some might argue that we have already established such a precedent with the LPN/LVN and the RN. The RN need not be an LPN before proceeding to RN education and licensure.

Of course, we are not starting from scratch in posing the generic model of advanced practice nursing; that would most assuredly limit our possibilities. The common definitions of advanced practice nursing acknowledge four categories: nurse anesthetist, nurse midwife, clinical nurse specialist, and nurse practitioner. They are now firmly embedded in our tradition and known to the public. It should also be acknowledged that some organizations, or minorities within them, would claim that generic advanced practice nursing does not exist; only nursing. However, the existence of separate legal status cannot be denied.

Thus we are faced with a pure model and a historical or modified general model. These three possibilities are diagrammed below.

Three Generic Models

Generic Advanced Practice Model:
ADVANCED PRACTICE NURSES

Modified or Historical or Definitional Generic
Advanced Practice Model:

NURSE ANESTHETISTS
NURSE MIDWIVES
CLINICAL NURSE SPECIALISTS
NURSE PRACTITIONERS

Further Modification of the Generic Model:
FUTURISTIC MODEL FOR ADVANCED PRACTICE REGISTERED NURSES

Specialty Models and Specialty/Subspecialty Mixed Models

Our current model could be defined by licensure or by certification. To define it by licensure, we would have to include the title of every advanced practice category in the 50 states. Similarly, to define it by certification, we would list the advanced practice titles issued by certifying bodies. We would be at a loss to construct a diagram.

Today's model is one of historical evolution, as nursing has responded to trends, demands, and opportunities as they have occurred. There have been efforts to distinguish between specialties and subspecialties. In the positions of a number of organizations we find a variety of attempts to make the distinction. It is interesting that, in struggling to arrive at workable definitions, some have resorted to the Nightingale tradition of defining what nursing is and what it is not. What is a broad (core) specialty and what is not?

As a reminder, among organizational samples we found the following:

▌ The National Council of State Boards of Nursing defines *specialty* as a broad, population-based focus of study encompassing common problems of that group of patients and likely comorbidities, interventions, and responses to those problems, e.g., neonatal, child, women, adult, family, mental health, anesthesia, and midwifery. [*Note*: These are *not* specific diseases or health problems or specific interventions.] The NCSBN likewise defines *subspecialty* as a focus of practice within a specialty, assuring expert knowledge of a particular area of patient problem, e.g., cardiovascular disease, palliative care, oncology, substance abuse, orthopedics, critical care, etc.

▌ The National Association of Clinical Nurse Specialists defines specialty focus as the client, population, type of problem, setting, type of care, and disease or medical specialty.

▌ The National Organization of Nurse Practitioner Faculties promotes broad categories of specialization within NP regulation (e.g., family, adult, gerontology, pediatric, women's health, psychiatric-mental health).

What is the defining concept or concepts whereby core specialties and subspecialties are distinguished from one another? The Texas BNE proposal, as previously described, intends that core specialties be based upon population. Yet in looking at the list it is difficult to find the defining characteristic of population. Others use the concept of role. And occasionally role and population are mixed. Of the four categories in advanced practice registered nursing, loosely speaking, two could be said to be identified by role, a third by population, and a fourth by treatment. It would challenge our creativity, therefore, to find a single defining concept.

Also the relationship of specialties to subspecialties has not been clearly identified. For example, are subspecialties subsets of one or more broad (core) specialties? If so, is certification in the core specialty prerequisite to certification in the subspecialty? And must both credentials be maintained for continued practice? Or are the core specialty and subspecialty examinations combined, e.g., core and modular certification? Ten years ago the ANCC studied the concept of core and modular certification: core for specialties, modular for subspecialties; core prerequisite to modular. And if the subspecialties are built on advanced practice cores, licensed to address public safety concerns, would there be reason to grant a special license for the subspecialty component?

The Missing Model

In reading the above, outsiders looking in on our profession might ask whether there is a pure generic nursing, as is the case in most professions. Do we have professionals and assistants or associates? Or do we have levels? Or are we a continuum of expanding scope of practice and competencies? If we search for the answer in organizational literature, we could be said to be one profession. If we search for the answer in licensing, we might infer that we practice at three levels—vocational nursing, registered nursing, and advanced practice—and that advanced practice begins at the RN level. This is our history. It must be carefully considered in reaching accord about the future. However, this is not to say that we cannot make fundamental changes.

And, if we are open to consider all possibilities, we must recognize the missing model, the one adopted by our "partners" in health care and other professions:

Modern Model of the Health Professions

PROFESSIONALS

Prepared at the graduate level

Licensed upon graduation

Some educated and certified as specialists

Assisting or associate or technical personnel in any number of categories

Making the Choice

By what processes are such areas now defined and approved? Boards of nursing approve areas for licensure. Certifying bodies—often at the urging or with the consent of specialty organizations—approve areas for certification. Accrediting bodies such as the ABNS and NCCA approve certification programs. Universities approve their graduate programs. State boards and national and regional bodies accredit or approve the schools. Many organizations have produced guidelines for defining specialties and subspecialties.

How is this pulled together so that it can be said that the profession is self-regulating, self-determining? In fact, there is currently no centralized decision making on the organization or configuration of nursing practice. Today's quandary and debate have made this very obvious. If we truly understand the importance of credentialing to profession-building, we must realize that the integrity of our professional structure is threatened. It must be reinforced with a standing, comprehensive system for making these decisions.

We need a unity model, a representative model, even a partnership, to bring us together. Unilateral decisions, tinkering with the contemporary configuration, even today's remedy will have no solid future without a process to sustain it. The stakeholders have already been identified. Let us hope that for these purposes they accept that what is at stake is the totality of the body and practice of nursing.

Summary

As a profession we have not systematically and uniformly established the divisions and subdivisions of our practice. However, they do exist, driven by demand and opportunity, and are effective in many ways. Within the past decade, with the acceleration of the advanced practice movement, we have been proliferating specialties and subspecialties.

Recent professional activities indicate we are aware that we are approaching chaos, with no clear distinctions among categories and no prevailing mechanism for bringing order to a potential catastrophe. It is in recognizing that we are in potential disarray, seriously inhibiting the profession's effectiveness, that we can turn this into an opportunity to build a solid foundation for future development. We all know what we have to do. We must all agree to one paradigm for specialty practice and credentialing, and it must include a vision for tomorrow and a plan for its achievement.

We shall be what we determine to be. That's empowerment.

References

American Association of Colleges of Nursing (AACN). (1996.) *The essentials of master's education for advanced practice nursing.* http://www.aacn.nche.edu/Education/pdf/MasEssentials96.pdf.

National Organization of Nurse Practitioner Faculties (NONPF). (1997 and 2002.) *Criteria for evaluation of nurse practitioner programs.* http://www.nonpf.org/evalcriteria2002.pdf.

Chapter 5

Afterthoughts on
a Styles Scenario

Margretta Madden Styles, EdD, RN, FAAN

This new book, with the help of the other authors, has sought to assess the progress of the nursing profession in developing specialty practice, to provide a framework for examining current issues in advanced practice registered nursing, and to propose principles and options for the future.

I cannot have spent a career embroiled in professional politics and more than 20 years studying nursing specialties and the credentialing of nurses and specialists in the United States and abroad without having some opinions with respect to the road to be taken. I have decided not to intersperse them throughout the previous chapter discussing models, but to set them apart as an afterthought for those who wish to know my opinions.

The Model

First, as to a model for advanced practice specialties and subspecialties, my approach would be to deal with the realities of the day, keeping in mind the ideal for the future. Building on 2005 with an eye toward 2020 would be the hallmark of a Styles Scenario.

How would this apply specifically to the models as outlined? My goal for 2020 is the purely generic model for the profession, with all nurses prepared at the graduate level. Initially many would arrive through a career ladder, but eventually all would enter from a liberal arts education. This would require an elaborate phasing-in process, e.g., grandfathering, time limits, and other transition mechanisms, so that neither practicing nurses nor the overall supply would suffer. Nurses would be licensed at graduation and titled by the graduate degree. Most nurses would pursue specialty practice and specialty certification, with no additional license required, since there would be but one scope of practice with substantially increased autonomy for all. Technicians, associates, and assistants would be part of the nurse workforce.

Back to the present. I further believe that the APRN movement will be the greatest impetus toward my 2020 goal of the purely generic model for the profession, particularly if we maintain a more general, role-focused model in licensure at this critical juncture. Therefore, to solidify today, with an eye on tomorrow, I would propose that we reserve advanced practice licensure for only the broadest categories. I would derive these roles from a combination of the four embedded in the definition of advanced practice registered nursing. These would be the core of advanced practice. Under such broad categories, especially the clinical nurse specialist and the nurse practitioner, all advanced practice registered nurses should fit and be titled and licensed as APRNs. Additionally, they would bear the specialty title conferred by their certification.

As a last resort, if it is impossible to reach agreement on licensing only the four broad roles, two proposals—those of NCSBN and NONPF—seem most promising in arriving at a compromise on core advanced practice specialties. NCSBN has proposed to define a specialty as "a broad population-based focus . . . encompassing common problems of that group . . . e.g., neonatal, child, women, adult, family, mental health, anesthesia, midwifery," and would exclude from the core category "a specific disease/health problem or specific intervention" (NCSBN 2007; https://www.ncsbn.org/156.htm). NONPF, in affirming that they promote broad categories of specialization within NP regulation, offers the examples of family, adult, gerontology, pediatric, women's health, psychiatric-mental health (NONPF 2002; http://www.nonpf.org/finalaug2002.pdf). There is great similarity between the two.

Licensing and certifying bodies could agree on expected competencies, confirmed through core (generic) examinations, common to all APRNs. Specialty and subspecialty modules could be additive in nature, requiring no confirmation in licensure. As is true today, nurses would bear legal titles and certification titles, both protected by credentialing mechanisms.

How do we arrive at, implement, and sustain the model to be built?

The Process

It is my firm conviction that the crux of empowering advanced practice is not in tinkering with or even remedying the current system, but in firmly establishing an all-encompassing, standing process for making decisions for and in the future.

I can anticipate the moans from readers upon the suggestion that a new nursing organization be created. And I might join them were it not for my ICN experiences. In that setting, in which the stakeholders were all of the nurses and nursing organizations of the world, I learned the huge effectiveness of single-purpose, streamlined mechanisms for developing international guidelines for a global profession. We are no less capable in the United States. So I venture forth accordingly.

For discussion purposes we might refer to the mechanism for credentialing nursing specialties as a representative council, because it should embody many of the characteristics of such a body. Because of the multiple stakeholders, the mission of the council and, frankly, past failures to achieve accord, a model observing the following terms should be considered:

- First and foremost, it should be bound by an explicit, agreed upon, common, single mission having to do with the designation and credentialing of specialties and specialists.
- Organizations represented should be the stakeholders mentioned throughout, principally those who participate directly in implementing specialty models through licensing, certification, and accreditation. Advisory or non-voting members could also be included.
- To be independent, as it must be, it should be freestanding, not subsidiary to any organization.
- To promote stability, it should be a permanent, not ad hoc, body with regular meetings and rules of procedure. Representatives should be well-informed officials of member organizations, able to speak for their constituents. They should serve for a specified term, not attend on a rotating basis.
- Mechanisms for promoting the binding nature of the decisions should be considered.

A foundation interested in strengthening the nursing profession should be eager to contribute funds to the creation of this instrument of empowerment.

On the agenda for one of the early meetings of the council could be the principles for a prototypic advanced practice nursing model, such as those outlined in chapter 4. But all should begin with a vision for the future. These first steps should lay a solid foundation for moving forward in unity.

Lift off to 2020!

References

National Council of State Boards of Nursing (NCSBN). (2007.) *Nurse licensure compact administrators.* https://www.ncsbn.org/156.htm.

National Organization of Nurse Practitioner Faculties (NONPF). (2002.) *Nurse practitioner primary care competencies in specialty areas: Adult, family, gerontological, pediatric and women's health.* http://www.nonpf.org/finalaug2002.pdf.

Appendix A

Certified Advanced Practice Registered Nurses: Role, Certification, Credential, Numbers, and Eligibility Criteria

Mary Jean Schumann, RN, MSN, MBA, CPNP

There have been dramatic increases in the numbers and specialty certifications of APRNs since the first (1989) edition of this book. Appendix A is an attempt to demonstrate both the growth in numbers of those certified as APRNs and the increasing requirements for preparation of those certified. This table provides a partial comparison of the qualifications for certification by credential and is a source for pursuit of further information about the eligibility requirements of each. The table is not exhaustive. Information is based upon the information that was available at printing and is attributed to those organizations granting the credentials cited. Exclusions are not meant to imply qualitative differences or acceptability of various credentials, but rather lack of availability. It is hoped that this table might become one that is periodically updated and made available under the auspices of the American Nurses Association.

All data was current as of January 1, 2007, the latest for which reliable data was available.

Certified APRNs: Role, Certification, Credential, Numbers, and Eligibility Criteria (Data current as of 01/01/07)

Role	Certification	Credential	Credential-Granting Organization	Numbers Ever Certified	Numbers Current and Active	Education Required	RN Licensure (active and current)	Minimum Master's-Level Education Required?	Additional Information
						Current Eligibility Criteria for Certification			
Nurse Anesthetist	Certified Registered Nurse Anesthetist	CRNA	National Board for Certification and Recertification of Nurse Anesthetists (NBCRNA)	55,368	33,856	Satisfactory completion of graduate nurse anesthesia program accredited by COA; comply with state requirements for current and unrestricted license as RN.	yes	yes	www.aana.com
Nurse Midwife	Certified Nurse Midwife	CNM	American Midwifery Certification Board (AMCB)	11,049	10,920	Satisfactory completion of a CNM accredited or with pre-accreditation status of a program in nurse midwifery (or in a Master's program satisfactory completion of all basic theoretical and clinical requirements of the nurse midwifery components.	yes	yes (by 2010)	www.amcbmidwife.org
Nurse Practitioner	Certified Pediatric Nurse Practitioner	CPNP	Pediatric Nursing Certification Board (PNCB)	12,163	9,955	Completed PNCB recognized Master-level NP program; documentation of current PNP clinical practice skills if longer than 24 months after completion of program.	yes	yes	www.pncb.org
Nurse Practitioner	Neonatal Nurse Practitioner	NNP	National Certification Corporation (NCC)	4,066	3,621	Satisfactory completion of Master's degree in specialty earned no earlier than 2005.	yes	yes	www.nccnet.org
Nurse Practitioner	Women's Health Care Nurse Practitioner	WHNP	National Certification Corporation (NCC)	12,530	10,038	Satisfactory completion of Master's degree in specialty earned no earlier than 2005.	yes	yes	www.nccnet.org
Nurse Practitioner	Advanced Diabetes Management Nurse Practitioner	APRN,BC,ADM	American Nurses Credentialing Center (ANCC)	Not Available	248	Hold licensure, registration and/or certification as a nurse practitioner. Within 48 months prior to application for this certification must complete a minimum of 500 hours in advanced diabetes management after licensure and/or certification as APRN. All requirements must be completed prior to application for certification.	yes	yes	www.nursecredentialing.org

	Specialty	Credential	Certifying Body		Number	Requirements			Website
Nurse Practitioner	Acute Care Nurse Practitioner	APRN,BC	American Nurses Credentialing Center (ANCC)	Not Available	4,638	Own a Master's, post-Master's, or doctorate from a nurse practitioner program accredited by CCNE or NLNAC in the same specialty as the certification. All requirements must be completed prior to application for certification.	yes	yes	www.nursecredentialing.org
Nurse Practitioner	Adult Nurse Practitioner	APRN,BC	American Nurses Credentialing Center (ANCC)	Not Available	15,345	Own a Master's, post-Master's, or doctorate from a nurse practitioner program accredited by CCNE or NLNAC in the same specialty as the certification. All requirements must be completed prior to application for certification.	yes	yes	www.nursecredentialing.org
Nurse Practitioner	Adult Psychiatric and Mental Health Nurse Practitioner	APRN,BC	American Nurses Credentialing Center (ANCC)	Not Available	1,581	Own a Master's, post-Master's, or doctorate from a nurse practitioner program accredited by CCNE or NLNAC in the same specialty as the certification. All requirements must be completed prior to application for certification.	yes	yes	www.nursecredentialing.org
Nurse Practitioner	Family Nurse Practitioner	APRN,BC	American Nurses Credentialing Center (ANCC)	Not Available	35,813	Own a Master's, post-Master's, or doctorate from a nurse practitioner program accredited by CCNE or NLNAC in the same specialty as the certification. All requirements must be completed prior to application for certification.	yes	yes	www.nursecredentialing.org
Nurse Practitioner	Family Psychiatric and Mental Health Nurse Practitioner	APRN,BC	American Nurses Credentialing Center (ANCC)	Not Available	530	Own a Master's, post-Master's, or doctorate from a nurse practitioner program accredited by CCNE or NLNAC in the same specialty as the certification. All requirements must be completed prior to application for certification.	yes	yes	www.nursecredentialing.org

Certified APRNs: Role, Certification, Credential, Numbers, and Eligibility Criteria (Data current as of 01/01/07)

Role	Certification	Credential	Credential-Granting Organization	Numbers Ever Certified	Numbers Current and Active	Current Eligibility Criteria for Certification — Education Required	RN Licensure (active and current)	Minimum Master's-Level Education Required?	Additional Information
Nurse Practitioner	Gerontological Nurse Practitioner	APRN,BC	American Nurses Credentialing Center (ANCC)	Not Available	3,704	Own a Master's, post-Master's, or doctorate from a nurse practitioner program accredited by CCNE or NLNAC in the same specialty as the certification. All requirements must be completed prior to application for certification.	yes	yes	www.nursecredentialing.org
Nurse Practitioner	Pediatric Nurse Practitioner	APRN,BC	American Nurses Credentialing Center (ANCC)	Not Available	2,964	Own a Master's, post-Master's, or doctorate from a nurse practitioner program accredited by CCNE or NLNAC in the same specialty as the certification. All requirements must be completed prior to application for certification.	yes	yes	www.nursecredentialing.org
Nurse Practitioner	School Nurse Practitioner	APRN,BC	American Nurses Credentialing Center (ANCC)	Not Available	96	Exam retired.	Not Available	Not Available	www.nursecredentialing.org
Nurse Practitioner	Adult Nurse Practitioner	NP-C	American Academy of Nurse Practitioners (AANP)	Not Available	4,775	Own a Master's, post-Master's, or doctorate from an approved nurse practitioner program in the same specialty as the certification. All requirements must be completed prior to sitting for the examination.	yes	yes	www.aanpcertification.org
Nurse Practitioner	Gerontological Nurse Practitioner	NP-C	American Academy of Nurse Practitioners Certification Programs (AANPCP)	Not Available	None	New exam 2007, first offering.	yes	yes	www.aanpcertification.org
Nurse Practitioner	Family Nurse Practitioner	NP-C	American Academy of Nurse Practitioners (AANP)	Not Available	14,325	Own a Master's, post-Master's, or doctorate from an approved nurse practitioner program in the same specialty as the certification. All requirements must be completed prior to sitting for the examination.	yes	yes	www.aanpcertification.org

Nurse Practitioner	Orthopedic Nurse Practitioner	ONP-C	Orthopedic Nurses Certification Board (ONCB)	Not Available	13	Satisfactory completion of Master's degree in nursing (through 2008 only, certificate-prepared Nurse practitioners will be eligible; after 2008, Master's degree required for all candidates). Plus, minimum 3 years as RN and 1500 advanced practice hours for current orthopedic nurse clinician; 2500 for non-orthopedic nurse clinician.	yes	yes	www.oncb.org
Advanced Practice Registered Nurse	Advanced Practice Registered Nurse, board Certified-Palliative Care Management	APRN,BC-PCM	National Board for Certification for Hospice and Palliative Nurses (NBCHPN)	Not Available	171	Credential will be retired 12/31/2009.	yes	yes	www.nbchpn.org
Nurse Practitioner	Advanced Certified Hospice and Palliative Care Nurse	ACHPN	National Board for Certification for Hospice and Palliative Nurses (NBCHPN)	Not Available	142	Own Master's or higher degree in nursing from an advanced palliative care accredited education program providing both didactic and a minimum of 500 hours of supervised advanced practice (specifically in palliative care) in the year prior to applying for certification or post-Master's certificate meeting the above or Master's, post-Master's or higher degree in nursing from an APRN program as either a CNS or NP with 500 hours of post-Master's advanced practice in providing palliative care (direct and/or indirect) in the year prior to applying for certification.	yes	yes	www.nbchpn.org
Nurse Practitioner	Advanced Oncology Nurse Practitioner	AOCNP	Oncology Nurses Certification Corporation (ONCC)	Not Available	495	Successful completion of an accredited nurse practitioner program and a minimum of 500 hours of supervised clinical practice as an oncology nurse practitioner, which may be obtained within the NP program or following graduation from the program.	yes	yes	www.oncc.org

Certified APRNs: Role, Certification, Credential, Numbers, and Eligibility Criteria (Data current as of 01/01/07)

Role	Certification	Credential	Credential-Granting Organization	Numbers Ever Certified	Numbers Current and Active	Current Eligibility Criteria for Certification			Additional Information
						Education Required	RN Licensure (active and current)	Minimum Master's-Level Education Required?	
Umbrella for advanced practice registered nurses in oncology	Advanced Oncology Certified Nurse	AOCN	Oncology Nurses Certification Corporation (ONCC)	3,955	1,224	Exam retired in 2004. For AOCN recertification those in good standing can renew certification with a minimum of 1,000 hours in advanced practice nursing role in oncology within the 48 months prior to application for recertification.			web.oncc.org
Nurse Practitioner	Acute Care Nurse Practitioner	ACNPC	American Association of Critical Care Nurses Certification Corporation	Not Applicable	New Exam	Newly instituted credential. Must be graduate of an accredited Master's program with a concentration as an acute care nurse practitioner and includes a minimum of 500 supervised clinical hours directly related to the knowledge and role components of the acute care NP.	yes	yes	www.aacn.org
Clinical Nurse Specialist	Clinical Nurse Specialist in Adult Health	APRN,BC	American Nurses Credentialing Center (ANCC)	Not Available	2,552	Own a Master's, post-Master's, or doctorate from a clinical nurse specialist program accredited by CCNE or NLNAC in the same specialty as the certification. All requirements must be completed prior to application for certification.	yes	yes	www.nursecredentialing.org
Clinical Nurse Specialist	Clinical Nurse Specialist in Adult Psychiatric and Mental Health Nursing	APRN,BC	American Nurses Credentialing Center (ANCC)	Not Available	6,963	Own a Master's, post-Master's, or doctorate from a clinical nurse specialist program accredited by CCNE or NLNAC in the same specialty as the certification. All requirements must be completed prior to application for certification.	yes	yes	www.nursecredentialing.org

Role	Credential	Certifying Body		Number	Requirements			Website
Clinical Nurse Specialist	Clinical Nurse Specialist in Advanced Diabetes Management	APRN,BC,ADM	American Nurses Credentialing Center (ANCC)	Not Available	151	Hold licensure, registration, and/or certification as a clinical nurse specialist. Within 48 months prior to application for this cerification must complete a minimum of 500 hours in advanced diabetes management after licensure and/or certification as APRN. All requirements must be completed prior to application for certification.	yes	yes	www.nursecredentialing.org
Clinical Nurse Specialist	Clinical Nurse Specialist in Child and Adolescent Mental Health Nursing	APRN,BC	American Nurses Credentialing Center (ANCC)	Not Available	1,000	Own a Master's, post-Master's, or doctorate from a clinical nurse specialist program accredited by CCNE or NLNAC in the same specialty as the certification. All requirements must be completed prior to application for certification.	yes	yes	www.nursecredentialing.org
Clinical Nurse Specialist	Clinical Nurse Specialist in Community Health Nursing	APRN,BC	American Nurses Credentialing Center (ANCC)	Not Available	499	Own a Master's, post-Master's, or doctorate from a clinical nurse specialist program accredited by CCNE or NLNAC in the same specialty as the certification. All requirements must be completed prior to application for certification.	yes	yes	www.nursecredentialing.org
Clinical Nurse Specialist	Clinical Nurse Specialist in Gerontological Nursing	APRN,BC	American Nurses Credentialing Center (ANCC)	Not Available	650	Own a Master's, post-Master's, or doctorate from a clinical nurse specialist program accredited by CCNE or NLNAC in the same specialty as the certification. All requirements must be completed prior to application for certification.	yes	yes	www.nursecredentialing.org
Clinical Nurse Specialist	Clinical Nurse Specialist in Home Health Nursing	APRN,BC	American Nurses Credentialing Center (ANCC)	Not Available	37	Exam retired in May 2005.	yes	yes	www.nursecredentialing.org
Clinical Nurse Specialist	Clinical Nurse Specialist in Pediatric Nursing	APRN,BC	American Nurses Credentialing Center (ANCC)	Not Available	114	Own a Master's, post-Master's, or doctorate from a clinical nurse specialist program accredited by CCNE or NLNAC in the same specialty as the certification. All requirements must be completed prior to application for certification.	yes	yes	www.nursecredentialing.org

Certified APRNs: Role, Certification, Credential, Numbers, and Eligibility Criteria (Data current as of 01/01/07)

Role	Certification	Credential	Credential-Granting Organization	Numbers Ever Certified	Numbers Current and Active	Current Eligibility Criteria for Certification			Additional Information
						Education Required	RN Licensure (active and current)	Minimum Master's-Level Education Required?	
Clinical Nurse Specialist	Orthopedic Clinical Nurse Specialist	OCNS-C	Orthopedic Nurses Certification Board	Not Available	13	Satisfactory completion of Master's degree in nursing. Plus, minimum 3 years as RN and 1,500 advanced practice hours for current Orthopedic nurse clinician; 2,500 for non-Orthopedic nurse clinician.	yes	yes	www.oncb.org
Clinical Nurse Specialist	Clinical Nurse Specialist in Adult	CCNS	American Association of Critical Care Nurses Certification Corporation	Not Available	561	Completion of a Master's program or higher program offered by an accredited college or university with a concentration as an acute care/critical care CNS. Completion of 500 hours in direct clinical practice within the program.	yes	yes	www.aacn.org
Clinical Nurse Specialist	Clinical Nurse Specialist in Pediatrics	CCNS	American Association of Critical Care Nurses Certification Corporation	Not Available	29	Completion of a Master's program or higher program offered by an accredited college or university with a concentration as an acute care/critical care CNS. Completion of 500 hours in direct clinical practice within the program.	yes	yes	www.aacn.org
Clinical Nurse Specialist	Clinical Nurse Specialist in Neonatal	CCNS	American Association of Critical Care Nurses Certification Corporation	Not Available	28	Completion of a Master's program or higher program offered by an accredited college or university with a concentration as an acute care/critical care CNS. Completion of 500 hours in direct clinical practice within the program.	yes	yes	www.aacn.org
Clinical Nurse Specialist	Advanced Oncology Clinical Nurse Specialist	AOCNS	Oncology Nursing Certification Board	Not Available	204	Completion of a graduate program with a minimum of 500 hours of supervised clinical practice in advanced practice role in oncology, which may be obtained within the graduate program or following graduation from the program.	yes	yes	www.oncc.org

Appendix B

Address to the National Nurses Stakeholder Meeting on Advanced Practice

(December 16, 2004)

Margretta Madden Styles, EdD, RN, FAAN

In December 2004, Dr. Margretta Styles addressed the national APRN stakeholder community at ANA headquarters in Silver Spring, Maryland. Her charge was to provide insight and a framework for discussion of a coordinated model for the regulation of APRNs. Gretta went further, though, delivering a charge to the participants and the larger nursing community. Her charge was that we challenge ourselves as nurses to look at a future-oriented model that would not only serve the profession both today and far into its future, but would also incorporate all aspects of regulation in a coordinated and efficient fashion. (She defined *regulation* as including education, accreditation, certification, and legal recognition.) The following are her slides from that presentation. In providing one framework for thinking about the future, it also urges us further to create one that can support a paradigm shift in our thinking rather than simply a band-aid approach to the current jumbled system.

APRN Consensus Process Work Group: Organizations Represented at the Work Group Meetings

American Academy of Nurse Practitioners Certification Program

American Association of Colleges of Nursing

American Association of Critical Care Nurses Certification Corporation

American Association of Nurse Anesthetists

American Board of Nursing Specialties

American College of Nurse-Midwives

American Nurses Association

American Nurses Credentialing Center

American Organization of Nurse Executives

American Psychiatric Nurses Association

Association of Faculties of Pediatric Nurse Practitioners

Commission on Collegiate Nursing Education

APRN Compact Administrators

Council on Accreditation of Nurse Anesthesia Educational Programs

National Association of Clinical Nurse Specialists

National Association of Nurse Practitioners in Women's Health, Council on Accreditation

National Certification Corporation

National Council of State Boards of Nursing

National League for Nursing Accrediting Commission

National Organization of Nurse Practitioner Faculties

Oncology Nursing Certification Corporation

Pediatric Nursing Certification Board

Wound, Ostomy and Continence Nursing Certification Board

DHHS, HRSA, Division of Nursing (*observer*)

**NATIONAL NURSES
STAKEHOLDER
MEETING ON
ADVANCED
PRACTICE**

December 16, 2004

Margretta Madden Styles, EdD, RN, FAAN

**Issues, Goals, And
Options:**

A FRAMEWORK FOR
DISCUSSION

Structure For The Session

▌ Overview of Specialization and Credentialing
▌ Advanced Practice Nursing Today: Definitions, Positions, Examples, Issues
▌ Shaping the Future of Advanced Nursing Practice

Objectives for the Session

▌ To discuss credentialing forms and interrelationships
▌ To review existing and proposed divisions/specialties
▌ To agree on assumptions/principles
▌ To agree on a model for defining advanced practice divisions/specialties for regulatory purposes
▌ To draft a process for determining future divisions

Overview

SPECIALIZATION AND
CREDENTIALING

Credentialing Definitions

- Credential
- Credentialing
- Diploma/Degree-Granting
- Licensure/Registration
- Certification
- Accreditation/Approval
- Recognition

Complementarities Among Credentialing Processes

Licensure Authorities May Recognize:

- National accreditation of schools for approval purposes
- Certification of advanced practice nurses
- Accreditation of certifying bodies

Certification Bodies Rely Upon:

- Accreditation of schools and programs
- Guidelines of licensing bodies

Accreditation Bodies Rely Upon:

- Licensing authority requirements
- Requirements of certifying bodies

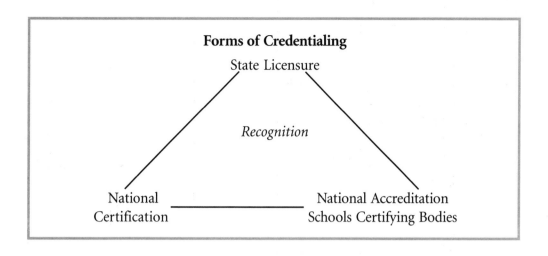

Forms of Credentialing

State Licensure

Recognition

National Certification   National Accreditation
                               Schools Certifying Bodies

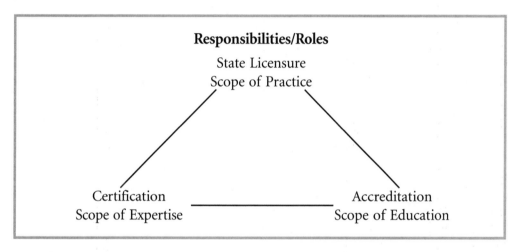

Responsibilities/Roles

State Licensure
Scope of Practice

Certification   Accreditation
Scope of Expertise   Scope of Education

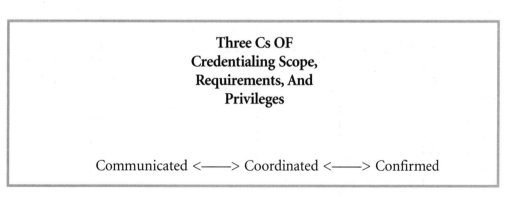

**Three Cs OF
Credentialing Scope,
Requirements, And
Privileges**

Communicated <——> Coordinated <——> Confirmed

Licensure—Determined by State Boards and NCSBN

- RN—generic scope of nursing, RN
- APRN—expanded practice privileges, APRN titles
  - Clinical Nurse Specialist
  - Nurse Practitioner
  - Nurse Anesthetist
  - Nurse Midwife

Certification—Determined by certifying bodies and parent organizations

- For RNs—covered by generic licensure
- For APRNs—advanced practice licenses necessary, if practice privileges extend beyond RN licensure

Accreditation—Determined by accreditation bodies and parent organizations

- RNs : Associate degree, diploma, baccalaureate programs
- APRNs : Master's and higher degree programs

ADVANCED PRACTICE SPECIALTIES TODAY

DEFINITIONS, POSITIONS, EXAMPLES, and ISSUES

*On Defining Specialties and
Subspecialties and Scope of
Practice for Credentialing
Purposes*
(Barbara Safriet)

National Council of State Boards of Nursing (NCSBN)

Specialty:

▌ A broad population-based focus of study encompassing common problems of that group of patients and likely co-morbidities, interventions, and responses to those problems.

▌ E.g., neonatal, child, women, adult, family, mental health, anesthesia, midwifery.

▌ NOT a specific disease/health problem or specific intervention.

NCSBN

Subspecialty:

▌ focus of practice within a specialty assuring expert knowledge of a particular area of patient problem; e.g., cardiovascular disease, palliative care, oncology, substance abuse, orthopedics, critical care, etc.

NCSBN

APRNs

▌ Masters preparation
▌ Program of study in a specialty area in an accredited nursing program
▌ Taking a licensing exam in same area
▌ Granted licensure in advanced practice
▌ Hallmark is direct patient care
▌ Subcategories: CRNA, CNM, NP, CNS

NCSBN

APRN Nursing

▌ Expanded scope which includes RN scope
▌ Scope includes advanced assessment, diagnosing, prescribing, selecting, administering, and dispensing therapeutic measures, including OTC, legend and controlled substances within the role and specialty-appropriate education and certification.

NCSBN

APRN Regulatory Principles

▌ Scope of education, certification, and practice are congruent.
▌ Role and title should reflect educational preparation and examination.
▌ APRN licensure is necessary because scope of practice exceeds RN scope.
▌ Boards must approve educational programs leading to licensure.

NCSBN

APRN Regulatory Principles

▌ Individuals must graduate from approved programs in the specialty
▌ Licensing exams must be acceptable to Boards of Nursing.
▌ Exams leading to licensure must be legally defensible and psychometrically sound.
▌ Content validity must be based on job analysis.
▌ All educational programs leading to licensure must be accredited.

NCSBN

APRN Regulatory Principles

▌ For dual track programs, each track must have a minimum of 500 clinical hours.
▌ The APRN specialty must consist of broad population-based focus of study.
▌ Curricula should be standardized and based on nationally recognized core competencies.

ANA Standards and Guidelines Committee (2004)

The profession of nursing has one scope of practice that encompasses the full range of nursing.

ANA Nursing's Social Policy Statement

Advanced practice registered nurses (that is, nurse practitioners, certified registered nurse anesthetists, certified nurse-midwives, and clinical nurse specialists) practice from both expanded and specialized knowledge and skills.

ANA Nursing Scope and Standards of Practice

Advanced practice registered nurses are RNs who have acquired advanced specialized clinical knowledge and skills to provide healthcare. As within all nursing practice, the level of expertise of the advanced practice nurse increases as they journey from novice to expert (Benner, 1982, p. 14)

American Association of Colleges of Nursing

The master's curriculum is conceptualized as having three components:

▌ Graduate Nursing Core: foundational curriculum content deemed essential for all students who pursue a master's degree in nursing regardless of specialty or functional focus.
▌ Advanced Practice Nursing Core: essential content to provide direct patient/ client services at an advanced level.
▌ Specialty Curriculum Content: those clinical and didacticllearning experiences identified and defined by the specialty nursing organizations.

National Association of Clinical Nurse Specialists (2004)

CNS Specialty Practice

▌ Specialty focus is the hallmark of CNS practice.
▌ CNS specialty is built on generalist preparation as an RN.
▌ CNS specialties may be broad or narrow, well established or emerging.

National Organization of Nurse Practitioner Faculties (2004)

1. Core preparation necessary to meet health care needs
2. Specialty preparation usually required for regulation
3. Subspecialty content value-added

NONPF and Regulation

NONPF promotes broad categories of specialization within NP regulation (e.g., family, adult, gerontology, pediatric, women's health, psychiatric-mental health).

▌ Allows more flexibility within the specialty practice area
▌ Allows for career mobility

American Nurses Credentialing Center (ANCC): Advanced Practice

Nurse Practitioners

1. Acute Care
2. Adult
3. Adult Psychiatric and Mental Health
4. Advanced Diabetes Management
5. Family
6. Family Psychiatric and Mental Health
7. Gerontological Nursing
8. Pediatric Nursing

American Nurses Credentialing Center (ANCC): Advanced Practice

Clinical Specialists

1. Advanced Diabetes Management
2. Adult Psychiatric–Mental Health
3. Child/Adolescent Psychiatric–Mental Health
4. Community Health
5. Gerontological Nursing
6. Home Health
7. Medical–Surgical
8. Pediatric Nursing

Texas BNE Proposal

Effective January 1, 2005, a registered nurse holding him or herself out to be an advanced practice nurse may be authorized to practice and hold a title in the following categories:

1. Nurse Anesthetist
2. Nurse Midwife

Texas BNE Proposal

3. Clinical Nurse Specialist in the following six specialties:
   a. Adult Health/Medical–Surgical Nursing
   b. Community Health Nursing
   c. Critical Care Nursing
   d. Gerontological Nursing
   e. Pediatric Nursing; and
   f. Psychiatric–Mental Health Nursing

Texas BNE Proposal

Nurse Practitioner in the following nine specialties:
a. Acute Care Adult
b. Acute Care Pediatric
c. Adult
d. Family
e. Gerontological
f. Neonatal
g. Pediatric
h. Psychiatric–Mental Health and/or
i. Women's Health

Responses to Texas Proposal

(selected and abbreviated)

Texas Nurses Association

▌ Unlike almost all other health care professionals, CNSs/NPs are currently regulated under what I characterize as a specialty-based model, i.e., the CNS/APN is recognized/licensed to practice in a specific specialty area and not simply as an APN or even as an NP or CNS.

Oncology Clinical Nurse Specialists (2004)

Specialization vs. Subspecialization

▌ Oncology meets the ABNS definition of a specialty and all related ABNS standards

▌ Examples of subspecialties within oncology:

1. Specific diseases or categories of diseases: leukemias, gynecologic cancers, CNS tumors, endocrine tumors
2. Specific treatment entities: blood and marrow transplantation, radiation oncology, surgical oncology

---

**Shaping The Future
Of Advanced Practice Nursing**

Models and Proposals for "Specialties and Subspecialties"

By what concept/defining characteristics are "broad areas" defined?

Models and Proposals for "Specialties and Subspecialties"

By what process are such areas defined and approved?

Shaping the Future Of Advanced Practice Nursing Options:

1. One core for all advanced practice nurses, NA, NM, CNS, NP
2. One core each for NA, NM, CNS, NP
3. One core each for NA, NM, CNS/NP
4. One core each for NA, NM, and broad areas of CNS and NP
5. Cores plus specialties/subspecialties
6. Specialties/subspecialties without core

Shaping the Future of Advanced Practice Nursing

Four Questions:

1. What goals/principles?
2. What model?
3. What concept?
4. What specialties?
5. What approval processes?

Question 1

What are the basic goals/principles that should characterize a credentialing system for Advanced Practice Nursing?

Question 2

What are the models that could be used for the system?

Question 3

What defining concept would be used for:

▌ Specialty?
▌ Subspecialty?

Question 4

What specialities and sub specialities would there be?

Question 5

What process might be used to move to a future model?

Appendix C

Nursing Specialization in 1989: The Text of On Specialization in Nursing: Toward a New Empowerment

Margretta Madden Styles, EdD, RN, FAAN

On Specialization in Nursing:
Toward a New Empowerment

Margretta M. Styles,
Ed.D., R.N., F.A.A.N.

Margretta M. Styles, Ed.D., R.N., F.A.A.N., is professor and holds the James P. and Marjorie A. Livingston Chair at the School of Nursing, University of California, San Francisco; she is immediate past president of the American Nurses' Association.

Published by

American Nurses' Foundation, Inc.
2420 Pershing Road
Kansas City, Missouri 64108

Contents

Preface and Acknowledgments

The American Nurses' Foundation (ANF) stimulated, sponsored, and supported this project by inviting me in 1983 to serve as Distinguished Scholar on any one of a range of subjects. I chose to pursue a study of specialization in nursing as best suited to my background and current interest. Previously, I had been privileged to chair the Committee for the Study of Credentialing in Nursing from 1977 to 1979, to serve on the National Commission on Nursing from 1980 to 1983, and to conduct the Project on the Regulation of Nursing for the International Council of Nurses from 1984 to 1985. Since 1985 I have been a member of the Board of Registered Nursing in California.

As an outgrowth of the above activities, I became convinced that specialty development and credentialing was an important frontier for the advancement of the profession. The ANF offered the inducement to explore that frontier.

The University of California, San Francisco (UCSF), augmented the material and human resources throughout the course of the project, as I moved in 1987 from being dean of the School of Nursing to being professor and holding the James P. and Marjorie A. Livingston Chair in Nursing. Patricia Struckman, J.D., administrative assistant, was particularly invaluable, providing services ranging from manuscript preparation to general project management.

Maryann Pranulis, D.N.Sc., R.N., clinical specialist in mental health and psychiatric nursing, served heroically as a UCSF postdoctoral fellow on the project. She conducted the literature review; collaborated in the conceptualization of the study, the design of instruments for data collection, and the development of the summary table of findings; and assisted in the first drafts of the earlier chapters. Dr. Pranulis left UCSF in 1986 to become associate chief, Nursing Service/Research at the Salt Lake City Veterans Administration Medical Center and assistant research professor at the University of Utah College of Nursing.

The American Nurses' Association and specialty organizations very generously contributed information to the study. And clinical specialists, who were captive audiences at a number of meetings attended by Dr. Pranulis, kindly served as convenience samples for our questionnaires.

I am immeasurably grateful to all of those who have helped in the production of this work. In many ways this project will be the capstone of my career in credentialing. I have long been fascinated with "the anatomy of a profession" and how the structure and function of professional subsystems and a dynamic environment influence the development and effectiveness of the total profession. I hope the recommendations rising out of this study will be accepted in the spirit in which they are offered, i.e., the burning desire to empower nursing to achieve its eminent destiny in the public interest.

MARGRETTA M. STYLES, ED.D., R.N., F.A.A.N.
Professor and Livingston Chair in Nursing
School of Nursing
University of California, San Francisco
  and
American Nurses' Foundation
  Distinguished Scholar
December 1988

Prologue:
Biological Metaphor

Philosopher and scientist Pierre Teilhard de Chardin applied natural law to social evolution in describing the humanization of the earth. Can his propositions be extended to the professional organism, that is, to the progress of nursing and other fields? Consider these passages from *The Phenomenon of Man* (1959).

First, Teilhard de Chardin described the general behaviors of isolated particles, i.e., *reproduction, multiplication, association,* and *controlled additivity.*

On *association* as a behavior of isolated particles, he observed:

In the first analysis . . . the grouping of living particles into complex organisms is an almost inevitable consequence of their multiplication (p. 106).

. . . association considered at all its levels, is not a sporadic or accidental appearance. . . . On the contrary, it represents one of the most universal and constant expedients (and thus one of the most significant) used by life in its expansion. Two of its advantages are immediately obvious. Thanks to it, living substance is able to build itself up in sufficient bulk to escape innumerable external obstacles . . . which paralyse the microscopic organisms. In biology, as in navigation, a certain size is physically necessary for certain movements. Thanks to it again, the organism (here too because of its increased volume) is able to find room inside itself to lodge the countless mechanisms *added successively* in the course of its differentiation (p. 107).

On *controlled additivity:*

The law of controlled complication, the mature stage of the process in which we get first the micro-molecule then the mega-molecule and finally the first cells, is known to biologists as *orthogenesis* (p. 108).

Without orthogenesis life would only have spread; with it there is an ascent of life that is invincible (p. 109).

From these elemental behaviors of isolated particles, Teilhard de Chardin progresses to describe four movements characterizing life at all levels and in all circumstances, *i.e.*, *groping profusion, constructive ingenuity, indifference, and global unity* (pp. 111–112).

As to *groping profusion:*

. . . the fundamental technique *of groping* [is] the specific and invincible weapon of all expanding multitudes. This groping strangely combines the blind fantasy of large numbers with the precise orientation of a specific target. It would be a mistake to see it as mere chance. Groping is *directed chance*. It means pervading everything so as to try everything, and trying everything so as to find everything. Surely in the last resort it is precisely to develop this procedure (always increasing in size and cost in proportion as it spreads) that nature has had recourse to profusion (p. 110).

On *indifference:*

[The] dramatic and perpetual opposition between the one born of the many and the many constantly born of the one runs through evolution (p. 111).

On *ingenuity*, the indispensable, constructive facet of additivity:

To accumulate characters in stable and coherent aggregates, life has to be very clever indeed. Not only has it to invent the machine but, like an engineer, so design it that it occupies the minimum space and is simple and resilient (p. 110).
What can be put together can be taken apart (p. 110).
By its very construction, it is true, every organism is always and inevitably reducible into its component parts. But it by no means follows that the sum of the parts is the same as the whole, or that, in the whole, some specifically new value may not emerge (p. 110).

On *global unity*, the embracing behavior of life at higher levels:

Though the proliferations of living matter are vast and manifold, they never lose their *solidarity*. A continuous adjustment coadapts them from without. A profound equilibrium gives them balance within (p. 112).

Evolution continues from these cells and levels to the whole of life (the aggregate) and its branches, through the stages of *ramification, aggregates of growth, maturity, socialization*, and *mutation*.

On the *ramification* of the living mass:

. . . let us study, over the whole extent of the living earth, the various movements whose aspect we have analysed in the instance of cells or groups of cells taken in isolation. Seen on such a huge scale one might well expect the multitude to be entangled in utter confusion. Or, inversely, we might expect that their total, in the process of harmonising, should create a continuous wave like the radiating ripple from a stone in a pool. But what actually happens is a third alternative. As we see it under our very eyes today, the "front" of advancing life is neither chaotic nor continuous. It is an aggregate of fragments at one and the same time divergent and arranged in tiers—classes, orders, families, genera, species (pp. 112–113).

Considered *as* a whole, life's advances go hand in hand with segmentation. As life expands, it splits spontaneously into large, natural, hierarchical units. It *ramifies* (p. 113).

On branches reaching for *maturity:*

The new invention, having reached the limit of its potentialities, enters its phase of conquest. Stronger now than its less perfected neighbours, the newly born group spreads and at the same time consolidates. It multiplies, but without further diversification. It has now entered its fully grown period and at the same time its period of stability (p. 116).

On *socialization,* the last touch to the phenomenon, the ultimate progress in consolidating and individualizing the extremities of its ramification:

. . . we find at the heart . . . a profound inclination towards socialisation. On the subject of socialisation . . . general observations [can be made] on the vital power of association. Since definite groupings of organised and differentiated individuals or aggregates (ants, bees, mankind) are relatively rare in nature, we might be tempted to think of them as freaks of evolution. But this early impression soon gives way to the opposite conviction—that they exemplify one of the most essential laws of organised matter. Is it the last resort employed by the living group to augment by mutual adherence its resistance to destruction and its capacity for conquest? Is it a useful means for increasing inner wealth by pooling resources? Whatever the fundamental reason may be, the fact is there: once they have attained their definitive form . . . the elements of a phylum tend to come together and form societies just as surely as the atoms of a solid body tend to crystallise (pp. 117–118).

Still change continues in the ramification of the living mass through the process *of mutation:*

. . . another pulsation of life surges, soon to divide in its turn . . . under the influence of the combined forces of aggregation and disjunction. A new phylum appears, grows, and spreads out above the branch on which it was born though without necessarily stifling or exhausting it. And so the process continues. Perhaps a third branch germinates on the second, and yet a fourth on the third—always provided the branches are on the right path and the general equilibrium of the biosphere is favourable (p. 118).

Teilhard de Chardin's final admonition on *beginnings* may apply to those who would undertake to study the specialization (the ramification) of professions:

Beginnings have an irritating but essential fragility, and one that should be taken to heart by all who occupy themselves with history.

It is the same *in every domain:* when anything really new begins to germinate around us, we cannot distinguish it—for the very good reason that it could only be recognised in the light of what it is going to be. Yet, if, when it has reached full growth, we look back to find its starting point, we only find that the starting point itself is now hidden from our view, destroyed or forgotten (p. 121).

Reference

Teilhard de Chardin, P. (1959). *Phenomenon of man* (B. Wall, Trans.). New York: Harper and Row, Publishers.

I. Introduction:
Background on the Project

Impetus for the Project

This project was initiated under the sponsorship of the American Nurses' Foundation (ANF) in 1983. In inaugurating its Distinguished Scholar program, the Foundation invited the author to study a critical issue confronting the profession and nominated "specialization" as one choice, known to be of interest to "the scholar," the American Nurses' Association (ANA), and nursing as a whole. Elaboration of the problem and methodology of the project were left solely to the discretion of the scholar.

Project Antecedents

From 1976 to 1979, the author chaired the Committee for the Study of Credentialing in Nursing, an independent body charged and funded by the ANA to assess and recommend future directions for credentialing[1] in nursing practice

---

1. Credentialing is herein defined as licensing, certification, registration, accreditation, and other "processes by which individuals or institutions, or one or more of their programs, are designated by a qualified agent as having met minimum standards at a specified time" (ANA, 1979, p. x).

and education. The study included the credentialing of specialists and proposed that specialists be voluntarily certified nationally within a free-standing credentialing center using standards established "by the professional society and professional specialty organizations as appropriate" (ANA, 1979, p. 88). The only standards specifically cited were "the credential for professional practice" as a prerequisite and mastery of "a body of knowledge and acquired skills in a particular specialty" (p. 88). No attempt was made to outline the boundaries of specialization or to identify particular specialties. A number of specialty organizations, as well as the ANA and other more broad-based associations, participated throughout the project as "cooperating groups" (pp. 94–95). Thus were born the author's interest in specialization, her familiarity with its controversies and dilemmas, and her respect for its structural and political nuances.

Concern for the growth, definition, and regulation of specialties as a developmental task as yet unfulfilled in nursing was heightened in 1983 as a result of two events. In the first place, the National Federation for Specialty Nursing Organizations, then a loose conglomerate of generalist and specialty groups, was proposing to incorporate, formalizing the status and relationships among the member associations. The Federation leadership kindly invited the author to speak to the assembly, analyzing the issues associated with this move. A major obstacle recognized in this effort to incorporate was that the specialties in the aggregate had no organized configuration nor uniform standards; therefore the definition of membership would be difficult.

Simultaneously, over a series of invited lectures around the country, the author was developing the concept of the "anatomy of the profession." Nursing's anatomy consisted of the divisions of knowledge and practice deduced from (1) the curricula of basic and graduate programs, (2) the content segments of examinations for RN licensure, (3) categories of certified specialists, (4) specialty organizations, and (5) job descriptions in the workplace. The proposition was advanced from cursory data that this structure was diffuse, diverse, unrecognizable, and potentially or theoretically, if not actually, dysfunctional (Styles, 1983).

The author's interest was engaged on an international level throughout 1984 when she conducted for the International Council of Nurses (ICN) a project on the regulation of nursing education and practice worldwide. The scope of the study included all categories of nursing personnel, generalists and specialists, basic and post-basic. Thus the problems and issues related to the specialization movement in the U.S.A. were viewed within a universe of similar developments and controversies around the globe. The ICN project culminated in a set of universal proposals to serve as the official ICN position on nursing regulation (ICN, 1985). Also, in 1986 the ANA published the first in its series on credentialing, a monograph by the author, comparing the status of American nursing to the guidelines proposed by ICN, including specialty regulation (Styles, 1986).

Objectives and Methods of the Project

In undertaking this project, the scholar's goals were to study, analyze, and propose. These have been achieved. Unfortunately, an original intent to include an historical, developmental perspective, identifying environmental influences, became unwieldy and unrealistic and had to be discarded.

The objectives, as they evolved with the project, were:

- To develop an analytic framework for examining nursing specialties,
- To study the characteristics of nursing specialties today,
- To analyze the characteristics of nursing specialties using the framework developed,
- To sample the opinions of nurses on specialty credentialing,
- To recommend future directions for specialization in nursing, and
- To prepare a monograph for publication by the ANF for the profession at large and the specialties.

Steps taken to achieve the above objectives were essentially: (1) a search for a conceptual framework in the literature of basic disciplines, (2) a review of the literature about specialization in general and nursing in particular, and of data from other studies and other informational materials, (3) development and administration of a questionnaire to elicit information from organizational representatives about identified specialties, (4) summarization of data about specialties, (5) analysis of data, using the conceptual framework to identify deficiencies, (6) development and administration of a questionnaire to elicit the opinions of convenience samples of nurses about specialty credentials, (7) compilation of the results of the opinion survey, and (8) formulation of recommendations to capitalize on strengths and to address deficiencies.

The conceptual framework is presented in Chapter II, the summary of nursing specialties today in Chapter III, the problem analysis in Chapter IV, indices of the relative power of specialty credentialing in nursing in Chapter V, the results of an opinion survey of nurses on specialty credentialing in Chapter VI, and recommendations for the future in Chapter VII.

Need for and Significance of the Project

Scholars and major study groups have pointed out the need for some regularization of nursing specialties. Hoeffer and Murphy in their 1984 monograph *Specialization in Nursing Practice* pointed out the need to establish consensus on nomenclature for practice roles for specialization and for credentialing of specialists (Hoeffer & Murphy, 1984). Williamson (1983), in analyzing the titles of graduate programs in nursing, identified a state of disorganization and inconsistency and, noting the need for consensus, called for "a national conference on graduate education and academic nomenclature" (p. 101).

In 1979 the Committee for the Study of Credentialing in Nursing reported lack of uniformity and fit in scope of specialty practice, lack of uniformity in requirements for certification, and minimal recognition of specialty certification in practice situations (ANA, 1979).

In the 1980 publication *Nursing: A Social Policy Statement,* the ANA acknowledged specialization as "a mark of the advancement of the nursing profession" (ANA, 1980, p. 21). The document proceeded to deal in a general way with developments in specialization and to articulate broad criteria for specialists. It spoke of emerging clusters of specialization and the responsibilities of universities and the ANA in these formative processes. While providing general direction, the statement, because of its very nature, stopped short of attempting to define established and emerging specialties.

Education for Nursing Practice in the Context of the 1980s (ANA, 1983), another important ANA publication reflecting the work of the National Task Force on Education for Nursing Practice, found that:

> No consistent or uniform mechanism exists at present to identify, classify, or otherwise control the various forms of preparation for advanced nursing practice. Moreover, just as nurses prepared in different entry-level programs are utilized similarly in practice, so are nurse specialists prepared in programs of different settings, focus, and length (p. 46).

The National Commission on Nursing (NCN, 1980–1983) recognized (1) rapid and uneven growth of specialization, (2) the emergence of a pluralistic system for standard setting as new organizations formed, and (3) the need for the profession to "specify the competency, accountability, education, and credentialing requirements [for clinical specialization]" (NCN, 1983, p. 15). The Commission called upon "the diverse nursing constituencies to join in formulating and supporting common policies in education, credentialing, and standards for practice" (p. 11). The 1983 Institute of Medicine (IOM) report *Nursing and Nursing Education: Public Policies and Private Actions* provided data illustrating the diffuse state of education and credentialing for nurses claiming to be clinical specialists and nurse practitioners (IOM, 1983, p. 139) and went on to support the need for more nurses prepared at the graduate level for clinical specialty practice (p. 140).

Using the methods outlined above, this study has undertaken to substantiate and address the needs recognized in these and other sources for bringing greater organization and rationality to the further development of the specialization movement in nursing, to strengthen it as a true "mark of the advancement of the nursing profession."

References

American Nurses' Association (1983). *Education for nursing practice in the context of the 1980s.* Kansas City, MO: Author.

American Nurses' Association (1980). *Nursing: A social policy statement.* Kansas City, MO: Author.

American Nurses' Association (1979). *The study of credentialing in nursing: A new approach* (Vol. I). Kansas City, MO: Author.

Hoeffer, B., & Murphy, S. A. (1984). *Specialization in nursing practice.* In I. L. Hirsch & R. V. Piemonte (Eds.), *Issues in professional nursing practice* (Monograph series). Kansas City, MO: American Nurses' Association.

Institute of Medicine (1983). *Nursing and nursing education: Public policies and private actions.* Washington, DC: National Academy Press.

International Council of Nurses (1985). *Report on the regulation of nursing.* Geneva: Author.

National Commission on Nursing (1983). *Summary report and recommendations.* Chicago, IL: Author.

Styles, M. (1983). Anatomy of a profession. *AORN, 38(3),* 484–498; *Rehabilitation Nursing,* 5(3), 10–13, 35; *Heart & Lung: The Journal of Critical Care, 12(6),* 570–575; *Nevada RNformation,* November, pp. 7, 14, 19.

Styles, M. (1986). *U.S.A. within a world view.* Monograph (No. G-172A) in series, *Credentialing in nursing: Contemporary developments and trends.* Kansas City, MO: American Nurses' Association.

Williamson, J. A. (1983). Master's education: A need for nomenclature. *Image: The Journal of Nursing Scholarship, 15(4),* 99–101.

II. Nursing as a Social System:
A Framework for Analysis

Search for a Conceptual Framework

What concepts or principles would best serve in the objective analysis of nursing specialization—its problems and possible solutions? A search was made to identify or create a conceptual framework to serve this purpose, the search initially sweeping widely through the disciplines of biology, philosophy, psychology, political science, economics, and sociology.

Philosopher-scientist Teilhard de Chardin's application of natural law to social evolution offered several tempting propositions from the biological analog, relating to the development, branching, and maturing of living organisms. His concepts are introduced in the Prologue to this report and are alluded to occasionally in the text in examining aspects of differentiation and specialism in the "professional organism."

In a 1986 comparison of approaches to the study of health professions, Dag Hofoss, a Norwegian health services researcher, reported how he looks at specialization from three different disciplines.

First, I assume the view of the sociologist (Specialization certainly is a reflection of the selfish interest of the professions, who strive for job monopoly), then, that of the physician (Specialization is the natural response to medical and technological progress) and, finally, that of the economist (Specialization is a result of increased market demand for health services) (Hofoss, p. 201).

He concluded that none of the three approaches is adequate in itself. The economic perspective, he argued, best explains the origin of specialties, since the specialization of the health professions is stimulated by rapid growth in the health sector. Thus, while specialization *cannot* resist the "pull of the market," it *can* begin in the absence of either professional initiatives or theoretical or technical advances (p. 205). Scientific and technological development and the deliberate efforts of the profession, as secondary factors in the development of specialization, influence its direction once begun. In Hofoss' opinion, the sociologist's view is most useful in examining the "profession-building" behavior of occupational subgroups, less as they originate than as they continue to evolve (p. 201).

During this trial and error search for a theoretical screen through which to examine specialization in nursing, it became apparent that professions are most appropriately viewed as dynamic social systems with political, psychological, economic, and legal forces operating upon and within them. Thus, an eclectic framework, suitable for problem analysis and proposal evaluation, was forged from elements of the sociology of work, social systems in general, and change theory. This chapter presents an overview of theoretical approaches relating to professions as dynamic social systems and then derives the framework for the study of specialization in nursing.

Overview of Methodological Approaches and Theoretical Orientations

In studying occupations, sociologists have examined the work, the worker, the work setting, and the occupation-at-large (Strauss, 1985). The phenomenon of specialization is pervasive and all-encompassing, as the work, workers, settings, and indeed the profession itself are organized to accommodate differentiated knowledge, skills, roles, and values. This project focuses broadly upon the profession-at-large, specifically upon characteristics defining developing and mature specialties and upon the relationships among specialties and between specialties and the total profession.

Occupations have been studied from historical, biographical, structural, and functional approaches. Nursing has been both selectively and comprehensively scrutinized as to significant events, trends, and people in its past. Seldom, however, have these developments been examined from a theoretical or analytic perspective.

Using a structural-functional-political backdrop, this study looks at a snapshot of the profession today as it has evolved with respect to specialization and therefrom considers and recommends directions for the future.

Social theory's main frame of reference is social action and interaction. Social relations progress from simple reciprocal, repeated interaction between social units to complex social systems of a higher order that are orderly, systematic, and enduring. Social systems are made up of structural elements and processes.

Structural elements within the social system include actors (participants), beliefs (knowledge), sentiment (feelings, values, and attitudes), goals or objectives (desired outcomes of work), norms (rules of behavior), status-role (position), rank (positional relationships), power (ability to influence the interaction), sanction (rule application), and facility (means).

Social system processes are of two classes, elemental and comprehensive. *Specialized elemental or functional processes,* such as knowledge development, tension management, role performance, and evaluation, articulate or express the functions of the separate elements. *Comprehensive master processes* bridge or integrate several or all of the elements and the social system and its environment. Master processes most important to the study of specialties and the profession-at-large are:

- **Communication**—transmission of thoughts and sentiment between and among actors,
- **Boundary maintenance**—establishing and maintaining the distinctions/division between and among the system's components and between the system's internal and external environments,
- **Systematic linkage**—establishing and maintaining connections between and among the elements,
- **Institutionalization**—internalizing a particular activity or element, rendering it identifiable as an integral part of the whole,
- **Socialization**—individual adoption of the values, norms, and identity of a particular role, and
- **Social control**—influence over the behavior of individual actors (Loomis & Loomis, 1961, pp. 15–17).

A functional systems orientation to the study of social systems, confined to the analysis of structures, boundaries, and functions or interactions, is useful for analyzing and describing the structural and functional characteristics of the profession as well as the specialty subsystems within it. However, as a singular approach, it has two limitations. First, it tends to define functional and dysfunctional systems in terms of equilibrium and disequilibrium, with adaptation or steady state considered to be functional. Secondly, this approach tends to inadequately address human behavior in terms of values and motivation and the power to bring about change.

Conflict theory adds a conflict-of-interest, psychological-political dimension to the above functional systems perspective, and introduces the following insights:

- Conflicts of interest are normal, inevitable, and ubiquitous in social relations.
- Some people in the social structure have more power and control over scarce resources than others, forming a power elite.
- Differential rewards accompany different roles to ensure an adequacy of trained, talented people.
- Once power is gained in one social sphere, there is usually an attempt to extend this influence to other spheres.
- Power must be legitimized (recognized as essential authority or source) in order to reduce challenges to that power.
- When power and legitimacy are used effectively, the structures are characterized by order, consensus, conformity, and integration.
- Although power structures are generally stable, they do not remain unchallenged or unchanged (Duke, 1976).

Conflict theory further acknowledges that the maintenance of power, once established, requires a set of conditions different from those used in acquiring power. *Power acquisition* is based on the competition for scarce resources model or, more pertinent to the study of occupations, the organizational necessity model. The *organizational necessity model*:

> ... presumes the existence of constant and natural tendencies toward increase in the size of social groups and the differentiation of structures and functions within such groups. This is congruent with a functional need for the creation of some roles or structures which will perform the task of coordinating the various roles and bringing all of the activities of the group into balance and integration with each other (Duke, 1976, p. 257).

Power maintenance depends on legitimacy, low conflict of interest, unity of social forces, low social change, and high homogeneity of people and values. It is also dependent on low levels of external threat and adequate levels of resources. Therefore, while the goal of the social system for functional theorists is equilibrium or adaptation, the goal for the "conflict" theorists is order, consensus, conformity, and integration—indices of effective use of power and legitimacy—and the system's ability to change without disintegration. A conflict theory orientation is useful in developing strategies to achieve structural and functional change.

Finally, from general systems theory it is important to note that social systems are open systems in constant interaction with the external environment. Open systems are dissipative structures that maintain their form and structure by continuously consuming energy.

The greater the complexity of the structure, the greater the consumption of energy and the greater the fluctuations within the system, with an increasing probability of reorganization into a new whole or evolution to a higher level of complexity (Ferguson, 1980; Prigogine, 1980).

Nursing as a Social System

So what does all of this mean for nursing and for this particular study? For purposes of examining the phenomenon of specialization, nursing is seen as a social system with structural elements and functional processes and internal and external boundaries. The external boundaries separate nursing from its environment; the internal boundaries define the specialties, each with its own structural elements and functional processes.

Structural Elements

Nursing-at-large is conceived as a social system composed of (a) specially educated and credentialed people (actors) with (b) shared values and expectations who (c) interact with each other and members of other health fields to (d) perform specific role functions (means) in (e) carrying out the work of the profession (goal).

The work of the profession, as defined by the American Nurses' Association in *Nursing: A Social Policy Statement* (1980), is to diagnose and treat human responses to health and illness. In Henderson's internationally recognized definition of nursing, the profession's primary function is:

> . . . to help persons, sick or well, from birth to death, with those activities of daily living that they would perform unaided if they had the strength, the will, and the knowledge. At the same time, and throughout this relationship, nurses help people to gain or regain independence and when independence is impossible, to cope with handicaps and irreversible disease, and finally to die with dignity when death is inevitable (Henderson, 1980, p. 246).

Such definitions establish nursing's external boundary and its relationship to other health professions. They also define nursing's goal as service to humankind to fulfill a need of society—a basic requirement of a professional discipline (Shermis, 1962).

Specialty Subsystems

As previously described, the organizational necessity model explains that social systems have a natural tendency to increase in complexity, i.e., to develop differentiated structures and functions, as they increase in size (Duke, 1976). Thus, in a large social system, such as a profession or occupation, when the work of the total system begins to expand, a la Hofoss' "the pull of the market," the profession begins to divide up the work of the whole and develop *specialty subsystems* in order to perform that work effectively.

As in the system-at-large, the specialty subsystems are also composed of the same *structural elements* as the whole: (1) actors (specialists), observing sanctions and organized by position and rank, (2) beliefs or knowledge, (3) systems of interaction, (4) goals, (5) means to achieve those goals, (6) values to drive the system, and (7) conditions and norms that limit the range of choices between and among goals and the available means. The specialty subsystems interact in concert to carry out the goal-directed work of the whole.

Functional Processes

In order to achieve the profession's goal of "diagnosing and treating responses to real and potential health problems," the profession-at-large, as well as its specialized subsystems, must conduct various functions, the means to goal attainment:

- **Practice**—carrying out the work of the profession, i.e., specified services to humankind,
- **Research and development**—generation and testing of knowledge and theory,
- **Education and socialization**—communication of knowledge, skills, values, and norms of behavior,
- **Standard-setting and credentialing**—setting and enforcing norms and standards, and
- **Organization**—conducting enabling functions, such as advocating and representing, defining the system's goals and boundaries, and gaining professional and public sanction.

Systematic Linkages Among the Functional Processes

The processes whereby the above functions are performed are systematically linked and the connections are maintained through communication and other integrating processes. For example, in the ideal situation, *research and development* first establish and test the knowledge base for *practice,* and, in order to be considered research of and for the profession, the research questions and the investigational approach must reflect the unique perspective (boundaries and values) of the profession (Donaldson & Crowley, 1978; Dickoff, James, & Wiedenbach, 1968). Second, the knowledge and skills, thus established, are communicated through *education* along with values and contribute to the efficiency or effectiveness of *practice.* Third, this knowledge/skill/value base is used as a foundation for establishing role functions and standards of performance by a *collective, organized body* representing the concerns of the profession. Fourth, the standards and role functions and substantive content derived from the knowledge base itself serve as criteria for *credentialing* potential practitioners for the whole of practice (licensure) and the specialties within it (cer-

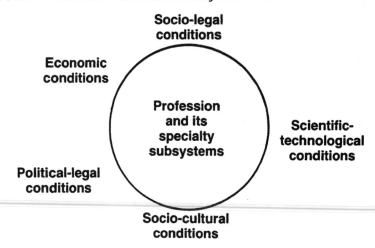

FIGURE 1 Environmental Conditions Influencing the Structure and Function of a Profession

tification).

When differentiated systems begin to emerge to carry out these functions, the systematic linkages between and among the functional systems must be deliberately established and maintained until they are self-sustaining.

External Influences

The complexification of a system is stimulated by the interaction between the internal and external environment. Within nursing's environment are conditions that may be classified as scientific-technological, socio-cultural, political-legal, and economic in nature. These conditions create either a *need* or an *opportunity* for the goal-directed activities of the profession or an *obstacle* to goal attainment, by controlling the availability of resources essential to maintain the system, as well as the market for the services of the profession and its specialty subsystems.

Environmental conditions must be favorable to enable the emergence of a new specialty or to allow for fluctuations within the system that will result in a viable, differentiated structure or function. Figure 1 reflects how these forces encircle the profession and its specialty subsystems, creating favorable or unfavorable conditions for change.

Summary

The conceptual framework for the study of nursing specialization was derived from a range of sociological theories, for the purpose of providing a basis for objective problem analysis and proposal development. This conceptualization of *nursing as a social system* consists of the structural elements, specialty subsystems, functions, systematic linkages, and external influences. Additionally, concepts from the conflict-of-interest approach to systems were introduced to provide insight into the dynamics of an evolving profession and its specialties and into the essentials for power acquisition and maintenance.

References

American Nurses' Association (1980). *Nursing: A social policy statement.* Kansas City, MO: Author.

Dickoff, J., James, P., & Wiedenbach, E. (1968). Theory in a practice discipline. *Nursing Research, 17(6),* 545–554.

Donaldson, S. K., & Crowley, D. M. (1978). The discipline of nursing. *Nursing Outlook, 26(2),* 113–120.

Duke, J. T. (1976). *Conflict and power in social life.* Provo, UT: Brigham Young University Press.

Ferguson, M. (1980). *The Aquarian conspiracy: Personal and social transformation in the 1980's.* Los Angeles: J. P. Tarcher, Inc.

Henderson, V. A. (1980). Preserving the essence of nursing in a technological age. *Journal of Advanced Nursing,* 5(3), 245–260.

Hofoss, D. (1986). Health professions: The origin of species. *Social Science and Medicine, 22(2),* 201–209.

Loomis, C. P., & Loomis, Z. K. (1961). *Modern social theories, selected American writers.* New York: D. Van Nostrand Company, Inc.

Prigogine, I. (1980). *From being to becoming.* San Francisco: W. H. Freeman Company.

Shermis, S. S. (1962). On becoming an intellectual discipline. *Phi Delta Kappan, 44,* 84–86.

Strauss, A. (1985). Work and the division of labor. *The Sociological Quarterly, 26(1),* 1–19.

III. Characteristics of Specialties in Nursing:
A Contemporary Survey

Introduction

What does a snapshot of nursing specialties today disclose? What are the specialties and how are they recognized? How are the specialties conducting their functions? Who are the nurse specialists and how are they qualified as specialists? This chapter attempts to answer these questions. A later chapter compares the power of specialty credentials in nursing to the power of specialty credentials in other health professions.

Identification of Specialties

The greatest challenge in the study of contemporary nursing specialization is the identification of the specialties themselves. Nursing has no single authoritative source for recognizing specialties, unlike other fields studied. Therefore, nursing specialties originate and are recognized in numerous and various ways, e.g., through educational programs, state "certification" or "second licensing" programs, national certification programs, specialty organizations and councils, and job descriptions. (The term "certification," when applied to state programs, is used throughout this report in a generic sense to refer to whatever mechanism the state governments use to recognize advanced practice.) As this survey has revealed, the aggregate of specialties designated via these sources is staggering in its size and complexity. Appendix A-1 (p. 70) includes a list of numerous specialty areas and specialties identified from three major sources:

▌ Graduate programs in nursing
▌ State "certification" programs
▌ National certification programs through ANA and other *certifying* bodies.

Also included as evidence of broad areas of practice are the councils of the American Nurses' Association (Appendix A-2, p. 102) and as evidence of newer developments, the standards of practice published by the ANA (Appendix A-3, p. 103). Overwhelming as this list may be, it is neither exhaustive nor current. New specialties and configurations and even new sources continue to proliferate. Moreover, identifying specialties designated through job descriptions would require a survey of every nursing service in this country. Specialization in nursing is a rapidly moving target for study, requiring a very fast lens for the scholar's camera.

Analyzing graduate program listings of the National League for Nursing (NLN, 1985) in order to determine patterns of specialization is very difficult. It is possible to count the frequency with which key words appear. However, the problem that arises is that these descriptors are in a variety of categories, such as diseases/pathology, systems, ages, settings, acuity, technologies or therapies, and functions or roles, and even subcategories for each. For example—

Diseases/pathology—oncology, diabetes, developmental disabilities, burns and trauma

Systems—cardiovascular, pulmonary, neurological, renal

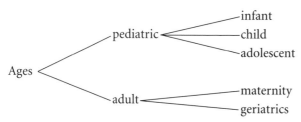

Acuity—emergency care, critical care, chronic illness, primary care

Settings—community, school

Technologies/therapies—anesthesia, IV therapy

Functions or roles—administration, teaching

Of course, these categories and examples are arguable and there are variants in any category by itself.

As the NLN list of graduate programs further discloses, because of the variety of categories, increased differentiation occurs through the grafting of one category to another. Any number of combinations is possible and even probable as proliferation continues. If this process continues unabated, in time a specialty or "sub-sub-subspecialty" may well develop in the administration of programs for geriatric patients with cancer of the gastrointestinal system who are receiving chemotherapy in the home.

Subspecialties are recognized phenomena in professions. However, the random development in nursing makes it difficult to ascertain which are the specialties and which are the subspecialties. There is no recognized hierarchy. For example, in pediatric oncology, does one specialize first in the care of children or in the care of patients with cancer? Is the disease or the age the broader category? Which is the stem and which is the branch? And does it make a difference? How can specialty certification program development accommodate to this lack of a conceptual schema for the evolution of nursing specialties?

How much consistency exists within state-recognized specialties is evidenced within the summary table in Appendix A-1 (p. 70). Nurse midwifery and nurse anesthesia are most common and less equivocal specialties because credentials beyond the RN are required for "entry" into specialty practice. The description "nurse practitioner" or "advanced practitioner" appears frequently as a broad category, occasionally qualified more narrowly as family, pediatric, adult, school health, mental health, etc. In some instances, "practitioner" recognition may be more closely related to title protection than practice restriction, the latter being the case with nurse midwives and anesthetists.

National certification is available through ANA and a number of nursing specialty boards (Appendix A-1, p. 70). One might expect that this quest to identify nursing specialties could be narrowed to the lists generated from national certification sources. However, this too is not as simple and definitive as it may seem. The ANA by its own acknowledgment offers generalist, practitioner, specialist, and administration certification programs, pointing out the definitional difficulties in differentiating among nurse generalists who practice in a specialized area, clinical nurse specialists, and nurse practitioners. Other specialty organizations have experienced these same difficulties in distinguishing "levels" or strata of specialty practice.

Three further problems with identifying specialties through national certification programs are that (1) some would seem to be subspecialties, (2) some appear to be overlapping, duplicative, even competitive, and (3) some true specialties may not as yet have developed certification programs.

How much consistency exists between and among the lists of graduate programs in nursing, state-recognized specialties, and national certification programs? Very little, because, as was mentioned earlier, hybridization is evident in graduate curricula; the state-recognized specialties are incomplete and generally quite broad; national certification has developed in large part parallel to the interests of specialty organizations; and there is no existing mechanism to coordinate these developments on the institutional, state, and federal levels.

The problem as described above in counting nursing specialties is reflected in the problem of counting nurse specialists. The aggregate number of certificate holders listed by the ANA and other national nursing certifying bodies is approximately 200,000 (American Board of Neuroscience Nursing, 1988; ANA, 1988). This figure is not synonymous with the number of nurses who identify as specialists through these and other means.

Survey of Selected National Specialties

Despite the fact that no definitive means has been found to identify nursing specialties as they exist today, a survey was carried out to determine how selected specialties are conducting their functions and how nurses qualify as specialists. This survey was completed in 1985 and must be seen as representing specialty nursing at that time only. ANA specialty and credentialing activities are reported in a separate segment of this chapter, because of the breadth of specialties and certifications encompassed within the organization.

Specialties included were those that had effectively self-identified as such through the creation of formal special-focus organizations, either independent or within parent associations. Some emerging groups may have escaped attention altogether or been recognized following completion of the survey. None was consciously omitted at the time of contact.

Initially all such specialty groups—identified and contacted under the auspices of the project sponsor, the American Nurses' Foundation—were asked to participate in the study by providing documents delineating their respective specialties and describing their membership. In response to this request, a total of 23 organizations furnished information, including brochures, position statements, articles of incorporation, bylaws, study reports, journals, and/or other materials. The documents were reviewed and the information organized and summarized.

To ensure the accuracy and comparability of the data and to elicit the most complete response possible, the process was carried a step further. Two survey tools were developed: (1) a summary table for each specialty and (2) guidelines for supplying information for such a table (Guidelines for Summary Description of Nursing Specialties). A blank survey table sample appears in Appendix A-4 (p. 105), and the associated guidelines in Appendix A-5 (p. 106).

A second request for participation was sent to all identified specialty groups. Those not responding to the initial contact were provided with a blank summary table and guidelines for its completion. Those who had supplied informational materials in response to the first invitation were provided with a completed summary table about their specialty and asked to verify and modify or augment the data contained therein. It was recognized that content overlap and cross membership may exist between specialty organizations, significant in itself in studying the specialization movement. No effort was made to determine the extent of dual or multiple membership. Overall, information has been collected on 23 specialties using the above-described procedures. The data collected are presented in table form in Appendix A-6 (p. 109).

Survey Framework

Problem analysis, as indicated in Chapter II on the conceptual framework, would revolve around a view of nursing as a social system. Therefore, the survey of specialties was designed to produce information about the pertinent elements of that system.

Nursing, in the aggregate and through its specialty subsystems, must conduct those functions necessary to achieve the profession's goal of "diagnosing and treating human responses to real and potential health problems" (ANA, 1980). Both specialized, functional processes (within the specialty subsystems) and comprehensive, master processes (binding the specialty subsystems to the whole of nursing) are essential to attainment of this goal. Thus, the survey of specialties attempted to determine if the means existed to conduct these specialized, functional processes and the bridging (master) processes.

Specifically, this called for the following data about each specialty subsystem:

1. **Master processes**—How does the subsystem (the specialty) relate to the total system (nursing)?
   a. Does it share the **goals** of the profession; i.e., is it a nursing specialty?
   b. Does it share the education and practice **standards** of the profession?
   c. What are its **structural ties** to the profession, i.e., formal relationships, communication linkages, etc.?
2. **Functional processes**—Through what means does the subsystem (the specialty) conduct its five basic internal functions?
   a. **Practice**—members (practitioners, specialists), roles, responsibilities, settings
   b. **Education**—programs for preparatory (basic), advanced, and continuing education
   c. **Research and development**—supportive mechanisms for development and dissemination of the knowledge base
   d. **Standard-setting and credentialing**—certification standards and procedures
   e. **Organization**—communication, representation, advocacy, and standard-setting mechanisms for enabling the above functions

Designed to supply answers to the above questions, the survey served as the basis for the ensuing general summary about nursing specialties today. Information regarding each "specialty" appears in Appendix A-6 (p. 109).

Major Characteristics of Specialties in Nursing

By 1985 nurses had formed more than 30 independent specialty organizations in the United States, in addition to numerous forums and councils in parent associations, to pursue their special interest areas (SIAs).

Identity and Focus

Do the "specialties" identify as nursing and in what manner do they divide up or organize the specialized work of the total profession? Does the use of master (bridging) processes by the SIAs vary? In what ways?

It was assumed that if a structure existed to conduct a functional process (e.g., if practice functions were defined), the specialty had at least minimal functional strength. Qualifying or quantifying functional strength or testing the assumption beyond this was not attempted in this project. To the extent that a wide range of performance or detail was apparent with respect to particular functions, some SIAs could be seen as more mature or better developed than others. In describing the more developed specialties, the word "mature" has been appropriated from Teilhard de Chardin's exposition of the evolutionary stages of social and biological systems and their branches. (See the Prologue.)

All but two of the specialty organizations participating in this project provided documentation of the special interest area's identification as "nursing." The SIA's identification as a *nursing* SIA was evident in the organization's definition of the SIA and its membership, the statement of purpose and goals, or the standards of practice. Two specialties that drew practitioners from a variety of backgrounds and disciplines in addition to nursing did not specifically identify themselves as "nursing." They were viewed as *nursing in specialty areas* rather than *nursing SIAs* and were not included in this analysis.

As evidenced in this self-identification process, specialties have organized around (1) roles, (2) loci or systems of care, (3) developmental stages of clients, (4) anatomical or functional systems or processes, and (5) diseases or pathology. Using this collapsed classification system, categorization was difficult in some instances and may well be challenged.

Practice

The majority of SIAs described the practitioner as a nurse, registered nurse, or professional nurse who provides nursing care to a selected population. Two SIAs described the practitioner as a "licensed nurse" or an "RN or LPN/LVN." Three SIAs defined more than one level of practice in a manner consistent with definitions put forth by the ANA in *Nursing: A Social Policy Statement* (ANA, 1980); these definitions differentiate between a generalist (or clinician) in a specialty area and a clinical nurse specialist. Two SIAs defined several role functions and levels of practice beyond those defined by ANA.

Definitions of functions (F), areas of responsibilities (R), and standards for practice (S) varied considerably among the SIAs. Only one SIA did not provide any information concerning F, R, and S. Several organizations reported that definitions of functions, areas of responsibility, and/or standards were in draft. Of those organizations with written and formalized definitions of functions, responsibilities, or standards, the definitions were developed either by the organization alone or in conjunction with the ANA. The scope and depth of the F, R, and S statements also varied, with some organizations defining only one of the three areas, others blending functions and responsibilities, and still others providing not only the standards but also the underlying scientific rationale for each standard. The presence and level of sophistication of the functions, responsibilities, and standards statements appeared to be an index of the degree of development of the organized special interest area.

As expected, the settings in which the SIAs were practiced also varied. SIAs concerning anatomical/functional systems/processes were more likely to be practiced in a variety of settings, whereas SIAs classified according to locus or system of care were practiced in fewer settings.

Education

Almost all of the SIAs required education as a "professional nurse" as the prerequisite educational base for practice in the SIA. However, only four specifically defined the baccalaureate in nursing as the entry requirement for professional practice and only one established a target date (1987) requiring the baccalaureate in nursing as a prerequisite for admission into specialty education. In the 1984 National Sample Survey (USDHHS, 1984), of the nearly 24,000 nurses who identified their principal position as "clinical nurse specialist," more than 11,000 did not hold a BSN or higher degree in nursing (p. 33).

In 1984 the ANA Council of Clinical Nurse Specialists conducted a survey of clinical nurse specialists who were members of state nurses' associations (ANA, 1986). Although this was not a representative sample of the total population of self-identified clinical nurse specialists in the United States, it is noteworthy because of the number of respondents (2,512) and the response rate of 74% (p. 1). In this study, 82% of the participants were master's prepared in their current specialty area (p. 51).

Recommendations and requirements for advanced preparation as a prerequisite for designation as a specialist varied. Some SIAs did not mandate advanced education, while the majority required either a certificate or a master's degree in the SIA for practice as a specialist. The availability of formal education programs in SIAs similarly varied from no programs to several graduate level programs. Three SIAs had established as a goal the phasing out of certificate programs and the movement toward incorporating their SIA education programs into master's or doctoral degree programs in nursing.

The availability and requirements for continuing education also varied. However, the majority of the organizations advocating or requiring continuing education were also providers of continuing education programs and were accredited as such by the ANA Regional Accrediting Committees. One SIA was also accredited by the ANA to approve SIA continuing education offerings. All of the organizations provided information about new techniques and procedures to their constituents through newsletters and/or journals.

The availability of a defined core curriculum also varied. Several organizations had developed and disseminated a core curriculum for SIA education, and two had developed curricular guidelines for defining which aspects of specialty content should be included in generic (pre-licensure) nursing education programs.

Because of the considerable variability, it appears that the educational characteristics are substantial indices of the maturity of the SIA. For example, the larger and more senior the SIA—

- The greater the likelihood that the SIA is in support of ANA's position on educational preparation for entry into professional practice,
- The greater the likelihood that advanced, formal education is required or proposed for practice as a specialist,
- The greater the likelihood that graduate level educational programs of study will be available in the SIA,
- The greater the likelihood that continuing education in the SIA will be a requirement,
- The greater the likelihood that the SIA organization will be an ANA-accredited provider of continuing education in nursing and will be accredited to approve SIA continuing education program offerings.

The availability of a standardized core curriculum was not consistently associated with other characteristics of practice or education.

Research and Development

All of the SIAs acknowledged the importance of research to the SIA knowledge-building. The majority had formed or were in the process of forming a research committee and had resources available to support SIA research. However, few held research symposia for the dissemination of current research findings. The organizations did hold research round tables, scientific exhibits, or research-based educational sessions at their annual meetings. One organization presented an annual award in recognition of outstanding nursing research.

The SIAs' knowledge bases varied considerably. Some cited advanced nursing theory along with knowledge derived from other disciplines as the SIA's knowledge base. Others indicated that their SIA knowledge was either based on the biological, medical, physical, or psychosocial sciences or a synthesis and application of knowledge derived from one or more basic or applied sciences. Three SIAs provided information about the specific concepts or areas of knowledge from other disciplines that were used to form their SIA knowledge base.

In a 1984 survey of clinical specialists completed by the ANA Council of Clinical Nurse Specialists, most respondents reported spending very little time in research and publication. They acknowledged, however, that a scientific nursing practice discipline is dependent upon theory building and empirical research studies (ANA, 1986, p. 53).

The identification, articulation, and development of the knowledge base are areas clearly requiring further attention. The functional system of research and development obviously requires higher priority in all of the SIAs, if specialty practice and nursing are to be better served.

Credentialing

All of the SIAs encouraged certification for specialty practice. The majority favored voluntary certification. School nursing deferred the certification process to state governments via the state departments of education, although the ANA recently established standards and a certification program for school nurses. Nurse anesthesia and nurse midwifery require certification by the Council on Certification of Nurse Anesthetists and the American College of Nurse-Midwives, respectively, as a prerequisite to specialty practice. Two of the SIAs did not have an established certification mechanism. All other SIAs had either set up an affiliated or independent certification board or recommended the certification programs of the ANA.

National voluntary certification through the profession was seen as highly desirable; in addition, state licensure was required for practice of several "specialties" in more than one state. Other forms of state regulation of advanced practice included state nurse practice acts, registration, authorization, notification of acceptability, and state recognition of certification by a duly authorized professional certification board (LaBar, 1983; NCSBN, 1988).

Criteria for certification varied, but all required clinical experience in the SIA. Only two specialties required satisfactory completion of an accredited specialty education program as a prerequisite. The certification procedures appeared to be uniform in the requirements for formal application and written examination. Only one level of certification was available even in SIAs recognizing that a distinction exists between generalists practicing in the specialty and clinical nurse specialists. One SIA required documentation of moral character and ethical conduct in addition to formal application and written examination. The clinical experience requirements for several SIAs were prohibitive for nurses employed on a part-time basis or whose primary role function is other than practice. However, some of the SIAs included hours spent in teaching, research, clinical administration, or SIA consultation toward the clinical experience qualifications.

Only two SIAs had, as yet, developed requirements and procedures for recertification. For nurse anesthetist recertification, the nurse was required to make formal application and provide evidence of state licensure to administer anesthesia and initial certification, evidence of 40 hours of continuing education in the previous two years, evidence of practice, and certification of personal/moral qualifications and conduct. Peer review was the procedure for recertification.

Because there is considerable variation in the SIA credentialing programs, it appears that the development of this functional system may be an indication of SIA progress. The more mature SIAs have developed rigorous criteria and procedures for certification and, in some instances, recertification. The number of nurses certified in 1988 by organizations outside the ANA is listed in Appendix A-7 (p. 155).

Organization

All of the nursing SIA organizations restricted full organizational membership to nurses practicing or teaching in that SIA. In some groups associate membership was extended to technicians, nonspecialty nurses, and other interested members of the health care field. All specialty organizations conducted annual business meetings, provided educational programs, published journals or newsletters, and defined or participated in defining standards of practice. Most had also established mechanisms and criteria for censure of members.

For several of the SIAs, the standards of practice also included organizational/institutional standards for enabling the practitioners' adherence to at least minimal performance. Thus, the SIA organizations were attempting to exert influence not only over the SIA practitioner but also over the settings in which they practiced. The majority of the organizations also indicated that they provided expert consultation or engaged in or contracted for lobbying for health care legislation concerning their SIA.

Publications

All of the SIA organizations published some type of periodical. The majority published newsletters to communicate information about the organization's activities, legislative concerns, and updates on new techniques, treatments, or procedures. Those organizations not publishing a separate newsletter incorporated this information into their journal publications.

Although all of the organizations published some type of journal, the content varied considerably, as did the nature and extent of peer review. The majority were clinically focused and included case vignettes, descriptions of new technologies, continuing education self-study modules, and editorials. Although research articles were included, few organizations had refereed journals devoted almost exclusively to research, such as *Heart and Lung*, the official journal of the American Association of Critical-Care Nurses. The extent and nature of the publications may well be an index of SIA functional development.

Relationships with Other Organizations and Disciplines

Most of the participating SIA organizations recognized the ANA as the official organization of nursing-at-large, as evidenced in their responses to specific questions regarding their relationship with ANA. Several groups also regarded the ANA as their lobbying agent. The majority indicated acceptance of and support for the ANA position on entry into practice and the social policy statement (ANA, 1980). However, they may not yet have incorporated these positions in their written documents. The majority also indicated that they engaged in joint ventures with the ANA or had provided consultation to the ANA in defining SIA concerns, standards of practice, and criteria for certification.

All of the participating SIA organizations were members of the National Federation for Specialty Nursing Organizations (NFSNO, Appendix A-8, p. 156) and/or the ANA-sponsored Nursing Organization Liaison Forum (NOLF, Appendix A-9, p. 157). The certifying agencies meet annually as the National Specialty Nursing Certifying Organizations (NSNCO), largely to exchange information and discuss issues of mutual concern. Thus, at least rudimentary efforts have been established between and among the organizations to work together as a "unified" whole in nursing. There was considerable variation in the number of other disciplines and agencies with which the SIAs communicated. Additionally, the nature of these relationships varied from SIA sponsorship to full collaborative efforts. These relationships, too, appear to be an indication of SIA development.

ANA Involvement in Specialization

The American Nurses' Association (ANA), the professional association for all nursing, also engages in nursing specialization activities, largely through its councils and credentialing programs. Therefore, a brief summary of related activities is included herein.

Five of ANA's functions directly related to specialization are (1) maintenance of specialty councils, (2) standard-setting for various practice areas, (3) nurse certification and recertification, (4) continuing education program accreditation, and (5) publication of a registry of certified nurses.

ANA councils, which individual members of state nurses' associations may join for an additional fee, are listed in Appendix A-2 (p. 102). Councils engage in various activities related to specialty practice, including promulgation of standards, policies, and positions; development of proposals for certification offerings and eligibility requirements; publication of newsletters; continuing education programming; and recognition of excellence in practice.

The ANA provides the most comprehensive and extensive certification program in nursing. Certification is offered in 19 areas within the broad categories of generalist certification, nurse practitioner certification, clinical specialist certification, and nursing administration certification. The ANA certification program schema appears in Appendix A-10 (p. 158). Appendix A-11 (p. 159) presents a summary of the requirements for the various ANA certification programs. The ANA currently requires the master's degree in nursing for certification as an advanced nursing administrator, clinical specialist in adult psychiatric and mental health nursing, and clinical specialist in medical-surgical nursing, and has declared its intent to raise the education standard to the master's degree in nursing for nurse practitioner certification by 1992. The ANA is also considering questions related to titling for the advanced nurse practitioner and clinical specialist.

Singly or in conjunction with other associations, the ANA has published practice standards in 22 specialty areas, as enumerated in Appendix A-3 (p. 103). The ANA accredits (1) direct providers of continuing education and (2) approvers of providers of continuing education, both for a period of four years.

In addition to the above specialty-related functions, the ANA serves as the administrator and convener of the Nursing Organization Liaison Forum (NOLF). NOLF is made up of 44 participating special interest organizations, many of which are associations for nurse specialists (Appendix A-9, p. 157).

ANA also recently inaugurated, with the support of a number of nursing certifying organizations, a *National Registry of Certified Nurses in Advanced Practice.* The purpose of the registry is "to provide for the public and the profession a national listing of nurse specialists and nurse practitioners who are certified in advanced practice by a national nursing certifying organization" (ANA, 1987, p. v). More specifically, the registry is intended to:

1. Provide listings of certified nurse specialists and certified nurse practitioners for use by the general public, voluntary and government agencies, insurers, employers, health care organizations, and health information and referral services.
2. Provide a means of identifying qualified individuals to serve on professional peer review panels.
3. Augment professional consultation and referral among nurses and other health care providers.
4. Increase accessibility and availability of nursing services for consumers (ANA, 1987, p. vii).

Summary and Conclusions

This chapter has painted in broad strokes a contemporary panorama of specialties in nursing. The difficulty in identifying specialties, as generated through a variety of sources, was presented. The results of a survey of selected specialties as to mechanisms for conducting the functional processes of nursing specialties and as to connections to nursing and health professions at large were reviewed. A voluminous appendix (Appendix A) presents the evidence upon which this survey chapter is based.

Information from 23 special interest area (SIA) organizations in nursing was reviewed, summarized, and analyzed in 1985 to determine the characteristics of emerging and mature SIAs in nursing and to determine which characteristics appeared to be related to the progress of the SIA as a mature specialty. The participating organizations represented all five major categories of SIAs identified for the study: roles, locus or system of care, developmental stage of the care recipient, anatomical or functional systems or processes, and diseases or pathology. Although the majority of the organizations had been formed since 1965, associations originating decades earlier also participated. Thus, there was a cross representation of "new" and "old" SIA organizations. The American Nurses' Association's activities in the realm of specialization and certification were reviewed and summarized separately.

The information provided by the participating organizations revealed notable differences in the existence and detail of the mechanisms for conducting the five specialized functional processes—practice, education, research and development, credentialing, and organization—as well as differences in the nature and scope of their publications and their relationships with other organizations and disciplines. Based on an analysis of the range of differences, it appears that the following characteristics could be acknowledged as composite indices of the developmental maturity of SIAs:

- **Practice.** The practitioner is defined as a professional nurse and differentiation is recognized (though perhaps not yet operationalized in certification) between a generalist in a specialty area and a master's-prepared clinical nurse specialist or practitioner. Functions, areas of responsibility, and standards of practice have been defined.
- **Education.** The baccalaureate in nursing is a prerequisite for entry into a formalized specialty education program, often at the graduate level, or it is the intent of the SIA to implement such a standard. Graduate level educational programs and continuing education programs in the specialty area are available (or emerging) and accredited by authoritative bodies. The SIA organization is accredited as a provider of continuing education and as an approver of continuing education programs.
- **Research and development.** There is visible support for and resources are directed toward research and knowledge-building in the SIA. The knowledge base has been identified, is empirically based, and is identifiable as advanced nursing knowledge. Research symposia are conducted regularly for the presentation of new research. Honorary recognition is awarded for outstanding research.
- **Credentialing.** A rigorous program of certification in the SIA is available with a procedure (or plan) for recertification.
- **Organization.** The concerns and interests of the SIA are represented by an organized body. The organization communicates with its members, carries forth the decisions, and represents the interests of the SIA to nursing-at-large and other groups or agencies as appropriate. The organization carries out studies pertinent to the concerns of the SIA, provides resources for the conduct of clinical research, conducts continuing education and research symposia, establishes

standards for practice and settings wherein the SIA is practiced, and has procedures and mechanisms for the extremes of commendation and censure.

▮ **Publications.** The SIA has refereed journals publishing SIA research. Other mechanisms are available for the regular communication of professional issues, information concerning legislation, new technologies and procedures, news of the organization, editorial opinion, etc.

▮ **Relationship with other organizations and disciplines.** The SIA recognizes the ANA as the official organization of nursing-at-large and enters into joint ventures with the ANA. The SIA maintains a communication link and cooperative efforts with other specialty organizations in nursing and pertinent agencies and organizations in other disciplines.

And finally, the SIA is identifiable as nursing through its definitions of practice and the practitioner, its educational programs and knowledge base, and its relationships with nursing-at-large.

It is a gratifying and inescapable conclusion that there is a great need and demand for nursing specialties and for nurse specialists. The emergence of specialty groups and certification programs, the number of nurses claiming specialization, and the vibrancy of the movement are all sources of strength for the profession. Subsequent chapters will consider whether and how that strength is to be channeled in the best interests of the public, the profession, and the nurse.

References

American Board of Neuroscience Nursing (1988). A directory of information on national specialty nursing certifying organizations and organizations planning to certify: November 1988 (mimeographed; available from American Board of Neuroscience Nursing, New York).

American Nurses' Association (1988). American Nurses' Association certification programs (mimeographed; available from ANA).

American Nurses' Association (1987). *National registry of certified nurses in advanced practice.* Kansas City, MO: Author.

American Nurses' Association (1986). *Clinical nurse specialists: Distribution and utilization.* Kansas City, MO: Author.

American Nurses' Association (1980). *Nursing: A social policy statement.* Kansas City, MO: Author.

LaBar, C. (1983). *The regulation of advanced nursing practice as provided for in nursing practice acts and administrative rules.* Kansas City, MO: American Nurses' Association.

National Council of State Boards of Nursing, Inc. (NCSBN, 1988). *Tabulated Data from the Advanced Practice Questionnaire.* (Available from author, Chicago, Illinois).

National League for Nursing (NLN, 1985). *Master's education in nursing: Route to opportunities in contemporary nursing 1985–1986.* New York: Author.

United States Department of Health and Human Services (USDHHS, 1986, June). *1984, the registered nurse population: Findings from the national sample survey of registered nurses* (No. HRP-0906938). Washington, DC: Author.

IV. Problem Analysis

Basis for Problem Analysis

The foundation for analyzing the phenomenon of specialization in nursing is made up of the theoretical framework derived for the study (Chapter II) and the summary of characteristics of specialization today (Chapter III). This chapter views those characteristics within the framework, addressing the central question: How does contemporary nursing measure up to the requirements for an effective, viable social system?

The following proposition, synthesized from social systems theory, serves as the basis for this analysis:

The nursing profession as a social system will be more or less functional to the extent that the functional processes within its specialty subsystems are adequate to contribute constructively to the work of the total profession and the comprehensive processes binding the total system are intact.

The profession will undergo the process of differentiation with integration to the extent that legitimacy, homogeneity, and unity, the conditions for power maintenance, exist.

This proposition incorporates several key concepts from social theory. The goals and components of a social system, in particular the interactive processes within and among subsystems, are examined from the structural-functional approach (Loomis & Loomis, 1961). From the perspective of social systems as dynamic entities within which conflicts of interest are being played out, the concept of power maintenance and the goal of system integration are borrowed (Duke, 1976).

Functional and Comprehensive Processes

What is a nursing specialty? Chapter III described how certification programs, specialty organizations, graduate programs, and standards of practice were searched in an attempt to identify nursing specialties. Countless "specialties" were derived in this manner. Information from 23 specialty organizations and the American Nurses' Association (ANA) was analyzed for evidence of the mechanisms for conducting the functional processes of practice, education, research and development, credentialing or sanction, and organization. Additionally, specialty linkages to the profession as a whole, through common goals and standards and structural ties, were examined. These processes are essential for nursing to achieve its mission with respect to the health of the nation and the self-actualization of its members.

Great variability was found among the specialties regarding the dimensions of practice and the development of its functional processes. Some specialties were found to be well-established, with explicit statements on scope of practice, roles, and curricula; graduate programs in the field; certification procedures; research support mechanisms; and large, vigorous organizations for pulling all of this together and moving forward in a systematic, unified manner. Others were found to be newer, less well-defined, and to be progressing tentatively. Ties to the profession as a whole are variable, with some specialties participating more actively than others in all-nursing or all-specialty organizations serving as means for setting standards and goals for nursing and for taking concerted action.

This variability is not surprising when nursing is seen as an evolving social system within a rapidly changing health care environment, rather than as a homeostatic system aggressively striving to maintain the status quo. However, such variability and flux add great importance to the conditions for power maintenance as this evolution occurs.

Conditions for Power Maintenance

Since nursing is a dynamic system of competing interests, specialization or differentiation can occur with system integration or disintegration. Integration, of course, is essential, if the profession is to survive and advance. What conditions are necessary for orderly change, for empowerment? A high degree of legitimacy, homogeneity, and unity (Duke, 1976).

Legitimacy

As viewed by social theorists cited in Chapter II, power must be legitimized (recognized as essential authority or source) in order to reduce challenges to that power. When power and legitimacy are used effectively, the structures are characterized by order, consensus, conformity, and integration (Duke, 1976).

Legitimacy is defined as "accordancy with law or accepted rules or principles." It is evident from the facts that nursing as a social system, in stark contrast to other professions, includes no single source of "accepted rules or principles" for the specialties, no means for external boundary-setting and sanction. There is no accepted authority for officially designating specialties and minimum specialty standards.

Legitimacy for the specialties emanates diffusely from (1) agencies certifying specialists—i.e., state governments, the ANA, and other organizations, (2) academic settings issuing degrees or certificates in specialties of their own design, (3) employment settings developing job descriptions for their own "specialists," and (4) governmental or other third-party payors at the federal and state levels agreeing to reimburse certain "specialists." The ANA has attempted to establish guidelines and set standards for specialties, singly and in concert with nursing specialty organizations, but must be seen to have limited recognition as an authority by the agencies of government, outside specialty groups, and employers who have established their separate definitions, processes, and standards. External powers, observing a lack of legitimation within the profession for its specialties, are free to define them in their own interests and to change or disregard those definitions as it pleases them.

Such absence of a source of legitimacy in the system leaves nursing-at-large, and the specialties themselves, susceptible to internal fluctuation and disorganization and especially vulnerable to outside forces competing for resources, equating to power, in the health care environment. Put quite simply, not only is there no decision on specialties, but there is no acknowledged place to decide where to decide. The profession and its members may choose instability and powerlessness deriving therefrom or may choose to confer the needed authority for specialties upon an existing or created agent they are willing to entrust with fairness in arbitrating conflicts of interest. Choosing the latter must reflect the belief that such arbitration and some degree of conformity are ultimately to the benefit of all.

Homogeneity

From the perspective of gaining and maintaining power by and within a dynamic system of special and competing interests, it is readily seen that some degree of homogeneity (consistency, equality, parity) is essential for the empowerment of each specialty and the total system. To acquire and hold their place in the system and for the system to undergo integrative change, specialties must seek comparability with respect to—

- Legitimacy,
- Definition and differentiation,
- Demand,
- Quality,
- Sanction,
- Stature,
- Representation and advocacy, and
- Structural and functional relationships (connectedness) to other parts of the system.

Legitimacy, or official sanction, has been discussed as a necessity for the total system to provide for its parts. Currently, specialties are operating without access or deference to professional legitimation, a failure of the profession as a whole. Once a formal means of establishing and enforcing broad guidelines for the specialties has been established by the profession, specialties could claim equal legitimacy as opposed to the current mode of self-recognition and random development.

Definition and differentiation are also an aspect of boundary-setting. Specialties must be able to describe, with equal clarity, exactly what special services are provided and how these contribute to the service goals of the total profession. If ill-defined, the specialty will not only falter in its development, but stands to be absorbed or squeezed out by stronger, newer interests, is open to challenge by other parts of the system, and may be in less demand or receive less recognition for its expert accomplishments.

Demand for services is another essential for maintaining power in a competitive environment. Therefore, for a specialty to earn the support of the profession, it must demonstrate that an insistent, enduring clientele exists and that this clientele is indeed the clientele of the total system; i.e., that these special services contribute to the overall practice of the profession.

Quality of services is a dimension of empowerment for the system and its subsystems. Specialties, wishing to be recognized, must strive to achieve the standards set by the profession and the most respected specialties. Indices of quality are educational standards, practice standards, certification and accreditation standards, and research productivity and dissemination. A specialty of lesser standards should anticipate a tenuous future within a fluctuating system.

Sanctions or credentialing processes are the major means through which quality standards are imposed. Certification procedures—at national, state, or institutional levels, permissive or mandatory—sanction practitioners. Accreditation procedures sanction programs preparing the practitioners. Specialties lacking such formal processes for quality control are at a disadvantage in seeking special recognition for expert services. Credentials must have a common meaning for specialties to gain parity and public recognition.

Stature, i.e., rank in the professional hierarchy, is necessary for a specialty to recruit, reward, and retain high caliber practitioners and to compete for influence and resources within the total system. Great diversity among specialty ranks leads to uneven quality and distribution of services and to member dissatisfaction, a chronic problem identified by all professions with respect to specialization. Thus it is essential that all specialties be highly valued.

Representation and advocacy mechanisms are essential for enabling specialties to aggregate, potentiate, and focus individual activity, to establish policy, and to provide a channel of communication and influence to the professional and external environment. Specialties lacking effective organization would be decidedly disadvantaged within a dynamic system of competing and often conflicting forces.

Structural and functional relationships to other parts of the system provide the avenue for reciprocal communication and influence. Through such means, credibility is established and the policies and future directions of the profession are shaped in its best interests and that of the public. Thus, each specialty should want the most effective connections to other specialties and the total system and its external environment. Isolation equates to impotency when interests within and external to nursing become very aggressive and conflictual.

Homogeneity is a mutual responsibility. To achieve orderly change and maintain power, the profession must promote a substantial degree of homogeneity with respect to legitimacy, definition, demand, quality, sanction, stature, advocacy, and connectedness among its specialties. The specialties, in turn, must develop the mechanisms to perform their internal functions and foster, utilize, influence, and conform to the mechanisms, processes, and specifications of the total profession. In nursing, the data indicate that the specialties have struggled valiantly and with variable success to organize and conduct their internal affairs as they have seen fit. However, to their disadvantage and the detriment of the profession as a whole, appropriate legitimacy and homogeneity have not been possible because the mechanisms to achieve these ends either have not been in place or have not been universally recognized as such.

Unity

Power maintenance within the environmental forces described in Chapter II requires a high degree of unity, i.e., accord, harmony, oneness. Within the total system, even as internal conflict and competition may rage, there must be unity of (1) purpose, (2) standards, and (3) fit among the subsystems. Unity does not imply stasis of purpose, standards, and fit, but a negotiated, dynamic order.

The total system is performing a service for the greater society. As to *purpose* or mission, there must be agreement as to the goal and nature of those services and the designated clientele. The ANA, through *Nursing: A Social Policy Statement* (1980), has attempted to describe nursing's purpose today. From what source do the specialties derive the overriding purpose of nursing and their particular services? To what overall purpose do they subscribe? Data from the study indicate a strong tendency toward recognition of a central purpose and a central authority for all nursing. However, some specialties have made this more explicit than others.

Where do the services of each specialty *fit* within the total range of services offered by the profession? It has been said that a high degree of definition and differentiation are essential for specialties. Does the profession provide a rationale for differentiation, i.e., a schema within which specialties can fit? The data show that nursing specialties have defined themselves by roles, loci or systems of care, developmental stages of client populations, anatomical or functional systems or processes, diseases or pathology, and technologies or therapies. Such random development could lead to an almost infinite variety of configurations of specialties and subspecialties and "sub-sub-sub-specialties." Without a rational, workable framework, unity of fit will be impossible, and overlap, competition, and confusion will result, weakening both the total system and its parts.

What *standards* best adhere to the overall goals of the profession? How are they established? And by what means are they enforced within the profession and its specialties? The data have disclosed great diversity in both the degree of specificity and the level of standards of education and practice, as reflected in position statements and certification requirements. As to education alone, specialty requirements range from short courses applied to any RN base to master's degrees in nursing built upon the BSN. A pattern seems to emerge suggesting differentiation between (1) those "generalists" practicing in a specialty and (2) clinical specialists, with the higher standard being applied to the latter. For some specialties this bi-level system is seen as a transitional phase until such time as all "specialists" are required to have graduate preparation in nursing.

The facts indicate that unity of purpose, standard, and fit are lacking, along with acknowledged mechanisms for their possible attainment.

Summary and Conclusions

Nursing's specialty development, when assessed according to the essentials of functional, integrative social systems, shows serious deficiencies. From the structural-functional perspective, an internal examination of the specialties discloses the variable degree to which the functions of practice, education, research and development, sanction/credentialing, and organization are performed, and equal variability in the maintenance of ties to the greater profession. From the dynamic perspective, it can be seen that the conditions for power maintenance—legitimacy or recognized authority, homogeneity, and unity—are grossly inadequate. While these deficiencies do not bode well for the future of the profession, they suggest ways for nursing to achieve specialization with integration and strength.

References

American Nurses' Association (1980). *Nursing: A social policy statement*. Kansas City, MO: Author.

Duke, J. T. (1976). *Conflict and power in social life.* Provo, UT: Brigham Young University Press.

Loomis, C. P., & Loomis, Z. K. (1961). *Modern social theories, selected American writers.* New York: D. Van Nostrand Company, Inc.

V. The Relative Power of Specialty Credentials in Nursing

CHAPTER CONTENTS

Introduction

Chapter IV, "Problem Analysis," hypothesized that nursing is weakened by the insufficiency of those conditions for power maintenance, i.e., the legitimacy or authority, homogeneity, and unity of its specialties. What is the evidence that this may or may not be true? To what extent do specialty credentials achieve the objective they are supposed to achieve?

Benefits of Specialization

Schnaps and Sales (1986), in a paper entitled "Specialization in Psychology: Lessons from Other Professions," traced specialization from the crafts and guilds of the Middle Ages to modern-day medicine, dentistry, nursing, law, and psychology. From a review of the literature, they identified several advantages to specialization in the professions having to do with (1) professional competence, (2) quality of services, (3) cost of services, and (4) professional satisfaction (Schnaps & Sales, 1986). Some of these benefits are summarized below.

Most fields have become too vast and complex for any one person to master the full range of information and skills encompassed within them. Specialization enables practitioners to concentrate in one area of knowledge and technique, contributing to the best possible services for clients with particular problems. It is argued that specialty standards and certification procedures lead to better prepared practitioners. Moreover, through the increased interaction of practitioners with similar preparation and interests, the exchange of ideas and discoveries is augmented.

Specialty certification is said to facilitate public recognition of practitioners with special qualifications and thus improve access to their expert care. Quality of services is also enhanced through external controls, for example, through having third-party payors link reimbursement to specialist certification. Schnaps and Sales also argued that efficiency, economies of scale, and cost-containment are possible through "standardized mass operations," and lend themselves to higher quality care.

Advantages of specialization to the practitioner are found to be both intrinsic and extrinsic in nature. Satisfaction often accompanies mastery of a branch of service and the ability to concentrate interests and energies, as well as the sense of close affiliation with a peer group. Increased professional stature accrues to specialists, along with increased income potential, although too many specialists may create underemployment. As was explained by Duke in Chapter II, differential rewards accompany different roles to ensure an adequacy of trained, talented people (Duke, 1976).

Indices of Empowerment

As to the above benefits of specialization, the question should be asked: How are specialty credentials in nursing recognized as a mark of professional competence, as an essential for quality control, as a tool for achieving efficiency and economy in managing health services, as a means of public communication, and as an avenue to professional satisfaction and reward? This chapter only poses some key indicators of specialty certification empowerment, each worthy of a study in itself. Anecdotal evidence appears below with respect to ten indices: professional identification, title and practice entitlements, institutional privileges, compensation, reimbursement, quality control, career advancement and recognition, recognition in nursing education, public awareness and consumer choice, and recruitment potential.

Professional Identification

As the data in Chapter III disclosed, the profession has no singular means of identifying specialists. Specialists are created by national certification, state "certification," graduate studies, employment job descriptions, and self-designation. Therefore, it is no surprise that in the modest survey conducted for this project (Chapter VI), while 86.4% of the respondents self-identified as specialists, only 46.2 percent claimed specialty certification. Certification is clearly not the definitive criterion for the nurse specialist. On the other hand, physicians' and dentists' claims to specialization are commonly understood to equate to board certification.

Title and Practice Entitlements

Certification in nursing seems to carry very limited extra practice entitlements. Title protection, more than expanded practice prerogatives, is the object of most state advanced practice legislation. Nurses certified by national voluntary agencies may use coveted initials behind their names. Exclusive practice privileges are largely confined to nurse midwives and nurse anesthetists.

Technicians are encroaching on nursing practice in some specialties. Legal and regulatory challenges to nurse specialists, largely from the medical profession, are often difficult to resolve, frequently requiring recourse to the scope of practice of the basic RN license and/or to restraint of trade protections.

Institutional Privileges

To what extent are institutional practice privileges expanded by specialty certification? Answering this question would require a survey of job descriptions. However, it is known that only a small minority of hospitals, 13% of those wherein nurses are represented by state nurses' associations, recognize specialty certification in salary scales (Collins, 1987, p. 39), and nurses have often indicated that such certification is not requisite to their positions (ANA, 1979; Collins, 1987). On the contrary, the practice privileges of physicians are very much determined by board certification. Nursing specialty credentials have clearly not been universally institutionalized in the structure and management of nursing services with the possible exception of the vast nursing enterprise of the Veterans Administration, where certification can lead to an advance of from one to five clinical and salary steps (USVA, 1983; Collins, 1987).

Compensation

The average net practice earnings of a general practitioner physician are about $75,000 per year, compared to $110,000 for those physicians certified in nonsurgical specialties and $150,000 for those certified in surgical specialties (Owens, 1987). The mean net income for general practice dentists is around $83,000, compared to $124,000 for dental specialists (ADA, 1986, p. 9). In 1987, the average salary for a clinical nurse specialist was about $4,000 higher (approximately 18%) than the average $21,700 salary for a staff nurse (ANA, 1987, p. 158).

In a 1985 article in *Dimensions of Critical Care Nursing,* Dunbar presented both sides of the debate as to whether certified nurses should receive a salary differential (Dunbar, 1985). That the question should be open for discussion is in itself a telling commentary on the benefits to specialty certification in nursing.

Reimbursement

Direct third-party reimbursement for nurses has long been an important goal within the nursing profession. In addition to being a source of independence and revenue to nurses, direct reimbursement has important cost, access, and quality implications for the public. As early as 1948, the American Nurses' Association had made third-party reimbursement for nursing services a priority. Some progress has been made since that time in securing such payments to nurses through social security, rural health clinics, and military dependent health programs legislation (Griffith, 1987). And several bills have been, and continue to be, introduced in Congress to expand the nursing services that would be covered. All of these legislative initiatives have sought third-party reimbursement for specialized nursing care of some sort, e.g., services of nurse practitioners, psychiatric/mental health specialists, perioperative nurses, midwives, etc. (Griffith, 1987).

Although progress in this effort has been very slow, the mere existence of the legislation underscores the potential for society's recognition of the nurse specialist as a professional health caregiver who provides distinct services worthy of distinct compensation. Nonetheless, nursing has far to go to achieve medicine's success in securing direct reimbursement.

Quality Control

Government regulations for the care of patients with a variety of illnesses, such as end stage renal disease, often specify the "board certified MD" as the caregiver. If there is any reference to nursing standards at all, the nebulous term "qualified or licensed nurses" is used. The most recent *Accreditation Manual for Hospitals* from the Joint Commission on Accreditation of Healthcare Organizations (JCAHO, 1988) gives recognition to many health profession specialists, but not to nurse specialists.

In describing the characteristics of the medical staff, the *Manual* notes that "specialty board certification is an excellent benchmark for the delineation of clinical privileges" and "such statements as the American College of Surgeons' *Statement on Qualifications for Surgical Privileges in Approved Hospitals* may also be useful" (JCAHO, 1988, p. 121).

Although the *Manual* does not require specialty certification for any medical staff, it does strongly recommend specialty certification as an appropriate and desirable criterion in selecting certain directors, physicians, and other hospital personnel, excluding nurses. It does *not* mention certification for nurses; instead it uses general and ambiguous terms such as "demonstrated" and "documented" to characterize competence. Nurse specialist credentials do not seem to be strongly associated with high quality service in the policies of regulatory agencies to the degree that this is true for other professions.

Career Advancement and Recognition

Nurse specialists have reported that many of their positions do not require certification and that they receive no special recognition for such. Intrinsic rewards are often cited as the only benefit to certification and thus possibly not worth the effort. Studies have found that the rewards of certification were largely intangible, including such nonmaterial rewards as the increase in personal satisfaction, the bolstering of self-esteem, and better working relations with nurse colleagues (ANA, 1979; Collins, 1987).

Recognition in Nursing Education

As was pointed out in Chapter III summarizing the characteristics of the specialties in nursing, the correspondence of graduate majors in nursing to specialty certification programs is very weak. In contrast, postgraduate medical and dental education closely parallel specialty board certification. Moreover, neither national voluntary accreditation nor state approval standards for schools of nursing require or endorse specialty certification for faculty teaching in prescribed clinical areas. Therefore, a potential for ensuring clinically competent teaching and supervision is largely untapped.

Public Awareness and Consumer Choice

Public understanding of what it means to be cared for by a physician specialist and specialists in other fields appears to be universal. On the other hand, consumers do not seem to think of nurses as specialists. One informal survey found that only 6% of the participants could name one nursing specialty (Kalisch, 1988). It seems unlikely, in view of these circumstances, that consumers can make informed choices about nursing care or that they will come to demand nurse specialists for their particular needs. Related access, cost savings, and quality benefits are thus being denied.

Recruitment Potential

How many recruitment ads and media spots feature certified nurse specialists and identify them as such? How many prospective recruits project themselves into a nursing specialty? The answers to these questions, too, are indications of the undeveloped power of specialty nursing credentials to attract the brightest and the best into the profession.

Summary and Conclusions

This chapter has introduced some clues to support the hypothesis that nursing specialty credentials lack the power to achieve the prospective benefits of specialization to the public, to nurses, and to the profession. The indices only touched upon herein represent fertile areas for further study. However, sufficient evidence is available to mandate that steps be taken by the profession to empower its specialties, lest they be further weakened by proliferation, encroachment, legal challenges, diminished status, and dwindling applicant pools.

References

American Dental Association Bureau of Economic and Behavioral Research (ADA, 1986). *The 1986 survey of dental practice: Income from the private practice of dentistry.* Chicago, IL: Author.

American Nurses' Association (ANA, 1987). *Facts about nursing 86–87.* Kansas City, MO: Author.

American Nurses' Association (ANA, 1979). *The study of credentialing in nursing: A new approach* (Vol. II). Kansas City, MO: Author.

Collins, H. L. (1987). Certification: Is the payoff worth the price? *RN*, pp. 36–44.

Duke, J. T. (1976). *Conflict and power in social life.* Provo, UT: Brigham Young University Press.

Dunbar, S. (1985). Should CCRN nurses receive a salary differential? *Dimensions of Critical Care Nursing, 4(6),* 361–367.

Griffith, H. M. (1987). Direct third party reimbursement for nursing service: A review of legislation and implementation. *Nursing Administration Quarterly, 12(1),* 19–23.

Joint Commission on Accreditation of Healthcare Organizations (JCAHO, 1988). *Accreditation manual for hospitals.* Chicago, IL: Author.

Kalisch, P. (1988, July). Personal communication.

Owens, A. (1987, September 7). Doctor's earnings: On the rise again. *Medical Economics*, pp. 212–237.

Schnaps, L. S., & Sales, B. (1986). *Specialization in psychology: Lessons from other professions.* Report to the Subcommittee on Specialization of the American Psychological Association's Board of Professional Affairs.

U.S. Veterans Administration (USVA, 1983). *Nurse VA qualification standards.* DM&S Supplement, MP-5, Part II, Chapter 2, Change 38, Appendix 2E.

VI. An Opinion Survey on Specialty Credentialing

CHAPTER CONTENTS

Introduction
Results

Introduction

What do nurses believe to be appropriate mechanisms and standards for specialty credentials? This information is important to know in considering recommendations for the future. For this reason, a sample survey was undertaken to begin to address this question.

In 1985–86, the author approached certain organizations to request permission to conduct a convenience sample opinion survey at one of their member meetings and/or conventions. Two organizations with broad-based memberships of generalist and specialist nurses, the National League for Nursing (NLN) and the Western Society of Research Nurses (WSRN), and two specialty organizations, the American Association of Critical-Care Nurses (AACN) and the Oncology Nursing Society (ONS), agreed to the distribution and collection of the survey questions and responses at their meetings.

The survey instrument included a range of questions about the respondents' status and their opinions about credentialing of nurse specialists, certifying bodies, educational programs, standards, and legitimacy. A sample of the opinion survey questionnaire is shown in Appendix B-1 (p. 166). A total of 286 nurses returned the survey questionnaire—111 from the NLN, 34 from the WSRN, 125 from AACN, and 16 from ONS. The information, as summarized below, is very limited in its generalizability because of the selective distribution of questionnaires and the small number of respondents. It is not known to what extent these opinions would apply to other groups or a larger population of nurses. Please see Appendix B-2 (p. 169) for a table of responses.

Results

When asked if they considered themselves to be specialists in a nursing practice area, 86.4% of the respondents indicated that they did. However, only 46.2% of the total said that they were certified in a specialty practice area. Nearly 65% of the AACN respondents were certified but only 12.5% of the oncology nurses were. Almost all of those who were certified reported that they were certified by a voluntary association rather than from a state licensing agency.

A series of questions was posed asking the respondents to order by rank a set of options for specialty credentialing. These included (1) no special credentialing, (2) education credential alone, (3) certification by voluntary association, (4) "certification" by state government, (5) certification by employers, and (6) certification by others. Forty-nine percent of the total respondents favored voluntary association certification as their first choice, and 38.1% gave top ranking to an education credential alone. Few respondents ranked state "certification" as a first option (6.3%) and only .7% (2 respondents) preferred employer certification.

The respondents were then asked which voluntary agency they would prefer to be the certifying body, choosing from (1) the American Nurses' Association, (2) nurse specialty organizations, (3) medical specialty organizations or an affiliate, (4) interdisciplinary specialty organizations, and (5) other. "A medical specialty organization or its affiliate" was not even ranked as an option by 86.6% of the respondents. Fifty percent of the aggregate chose the nurse specialty organization as the desirable agency for specialty certification; 45% and 47.1% of respondents from the broad-based NLN and WSRN groups, respectively, ranked certification by the ANA as the preferred choice; respondents from the two specialty organizations (AACN and ONS) ranked nurse specialty organization certification as the number one option (68% and 62.5% respectively).

Respondents were asked who should approve/accredit educational programs preparing for specialty practice. Choices were (1) NLN master's degree program accreditation, (2) NLN specialty program accreditation (currently not available), (3) ANA, (4) a body certifying the specialist, (5) state government (e.g., board of nursing), and (6) others. Thirty-six percent of the aggregate favored the body certifying the specialist as the program accreditor. Top choices by group were: 29.7% of the NLN respondents selected NLN master's program accreditation, 23.5% of WSRN respondents selected ANA, and 52.8% of AACN and 31.3% of ONS respondents, respectively, selected the specialist certifying body.

When questioned about who should set the standards for specialist certification, 52.1% of all respondents favored the nursing specialty organization as the appropriate body. This was the first choice of 67.2% and 56.3% of the AACN and ONS respondents, respectively. Fifty-three percent of the WSRN respondents favored the specialty bodies (councils) of the American Nurses' Association in this role. Of the NLN group, 50.4% selected either the ANA or its specialty councils. Again, state government was ranked very low in this capacity.

Regarding education, the respondents were asked what they would favor as the education standards for specialty practice/certification. They were offered choices for a prerequisite education base before specialty preparation that included (1) a BSN, (2) an AD or diploma, (3) any one of the three, and (4) other. Seventy-six percent of the aggregate chose the BSN as a prerequisite. When asked to then select preferred preparation for specialty practice, 61.2% of the aggregate chose the master's in nursing as the desirable educational program, while only 19.2% chose a nondegree certificate program. The master's degree was the emphatic choice for NLN and WSRN participants (71.2% and 88.2%), but it was less so for the AACN and ONS participants (47.2% and 43.8%).

Three different sets of options concerning certification policies/practices were then offered to the respondents. They were first asked (Option A) if they preferred certification for generalists practicing in a specialty area or certification for nurses prepared as specialists or both. Slightly more than 55% chose the "nurses prepared as specialists" option.

Option B asked whether they would prefer one level of certification for each specialty, or bi-level or multilevel certification for some specialties. In the aggregate 47.2% selected one level, 39.5% more than one level. Among AACN respondents, 48.8% favored the multilevel. Finally, in the third option (Option C), they were asked whether certification should be by broad areas of specialization only or whether there should be certification for specialties and subspecialties in some fields. The majority favored the latter choice, i.e., specialties and subspecialties. It should be noted, however, that between 11% and 44% of the respondents did not respond to the Options B and C questions, perhaps because they were somewhat confused by the use of the word "option."

In the final question, the respondents were asked to rank the importance of each of a list of factors in assessing the legitimacy of a proposed or emerging nursing specialty. They could answer "not important," "somewhat important," "very important," and "of critical importance." As can be seen below, in the aggregate the respondents found all of the factors, with the exception of the "government credentialing/certification required," to be either very important or of critical importance.

Identifiable as nursing
    Very important   12.9%
    Of critical importance   83.2%
Recognized by an authoritative body in nursing
    Very important   26.9%
    Of critical importance   62.6%

Highly developed empirical knowledge base
    Very important   42.6%
    Of critical importance   49.0%
Evidence that substantial human and other resources are devoted to research
    Very important   55.9%
    Of critical importance   27.3%
Published research concerning the specialty's knowledge base
    Very important   44.4%
    Of critical importance   37.8%
Refereed research journals devoted to the specialty's knowledge base
    Very important   43.3%
    Of critical importance   29.0%
Research conferences/symposia devoted to the specialty knowledge base
    Very important   44.7%
    Of critical importance   35.7%
Requires special skills, techniques, or technology
    Very important   25.1%
    Of critical importance   66.1%
Knowledge/skill base *not* included in generic education
    Very important   31.5%
    Of critical importance   32.5%
Specialty-education programs exist
    Very important   32.5%
    Of critical importance   55.6%
Requires graduate level education (master's or doctorate)
    Very important   27.9%
    Of critical importance   41.3%
Education program requires supervised clinical experience
    Very important   28.6%
    Of critical importance   58.4%
Specialists involved in establishing guidelines, criteria and/or mechanisms for
  credentialing
    Very important   23.4%
    Of critical importance   71.3%
Voluntary certification programs exist
    Very important   36.7%
    Of critical importance   38.5%
Government credentialing/certification required
    Not important   45.1%
    Somewhat important   31.4%
Independent specialty organization (or branch within another organization) exists
    Very important   36.7%
    Of critical importance   23.8%

Voting membership in the organization restricted to nurse specialists
    Very important   31.1%
    Of critical importance   22.4%
Specialty organization establishes practice and education standards
    Very important   29.7%
    Of critical importance   60.1%
Specialty organization provides mechanisms for maintaining quality research, education, and service
    Very important   28.7%
    Of critical importance   61.2%
Large and universal client population requiring specialized care
    Very important   42.7%
    Of critical importance   35.3%
Uniform practice standards
    Very important   37.1%
    Of critical importance   52.1%
Uniform role functions
    Very important   40.6%
    Of critical importance   30.1%
Uniform qualifications as prerequisites for practice
    Very important   38.4%
    Of critical importance   51.7%

VII. Proposals for Empowering Nursing as a Specialized Profession

The Essentials for Empowerment

The need for nurse specialists has multiplied with the magnitude and complexity of the health care system. Nurses and organizations have responded heroically to that demand, as the dramatic growth of specialties and specialists clearly attests. The challenge is to channel specialization constructively to the benefit of the public and the profession and the practitioner.

As identified in the problem analysis derived from social science theory (Chapter IV), nursing needs to achieve greater authority, homogeneity, and unity of its specialty subsystems if it is to attain its goals as a profession. Based on this analysis, there would seem to be four essentials for empowering nursing as a specialized social system:

I An authoritative, criterion-based professional review mechanism for specialty recognition and sanction.
I Criteria for accomplishing an adequate degree of homogeneity and ensuring specialty services of high quality.
I A schema within which unity of purpose and fit among the specialties can be determined.
I A plan for promoting specialist credentials.

This final chapter presents skeletal proposals for addressing these needs and concludes with recommendations for the review and implementation of the proposals.

A Mechanism for Specialty Approval

Making the crucial decision as to what constitutes a legitimate specialty in nursing and as to what specialties qualify is long overdue. The controversy and the challenge lie in designating or developing the authority for this process. Multiple parties are interested in such processes: the professional association; the education, certifying, accreditation, licensing, and service sectors; health care consumers; and, unquestionably, the specialties and specialists themselves.

The medical profession has frankly recognized all of these interests through an elaborate system of interlocking organizations. Policies and specialties are approved jointly by the American Medical Association (AMA) and the American Board of Medical Specialties (ABMS). The ABMS, created more than 50 years ago, is made up of member boards and national organizations concerned with graduate and continuing medical education and specialty practice, and public members. The primary function of the ABMS is "to assist members in their efforts to promote the quality and efficiency of the process of evaluating and certifying physician specialists" (ABMS, 1987, p. v). Residency programs preparing medical specialists are reviewed and approved by both the Accreditation Council for Graduate Medical Education and the Residency Review Committees (RRCs) for each of the medical specialties (ACGME, 1987).

The American Dental Association has recognized areas of specialty practice since 1940. Each of these specialties has established Boards that operate in accordance with American Dental Association requirements (ADA, 1986). These Boards set examination requirements and standards, appraise the qualifications of applicants, administer comprehensive examinations, and issue certification to those who qualify as diplomates (ADA, p. 1333). Eight specialties have been identified in this manner—dental public health, endodontics, oral pathology, oral and maxillofacial surgery, orthodontics, pedodontics, periodontics, and prosthodontics (ADA, 1982). Advanced educational programs can be offered either at the graduate level, leading to a master's or doctoral degree, or on a postgraduate basis, leading to a certification of completion (Call, 1987).

Pharmacy, on the other hand, has come late to specialization. However, from the beginning in 1976, the American Pharmaceutical Association (APhA) created *one* board, the Board of Pharmaceutical Specialties (BPS), with the authority to designate specialties and certify specialists (Zellmer, 1986). The APhA appoints to this Board six pharmacists, one physician, one nurse, and one public member (Penna, 1988). The Board recognized that "the *sine qua non* in establishing differential credentials is measured proficiency" (Walton, 1986).

Compared with other professions, nursing is in the anomalous situation of having multiple and diverse specialty authorities and certifying agencies, including its multipurpose, all-profession, parent organization, the American Nurses' Association (ANA). Other professions have tended to certify specialists within or outside of the professional association, but not both. And, when certification occurs outside of the association, close ties to the association have been maintained for coordination and standard-setting.

In making recommendations for providing an adequate degree of authority, homogeneity, and unity to specialty development, one can choose to accept and capitalize upon nursing's peculiarities or to rectify them. The former option, i.e., facing the present realities, with a goal of consistently high quality specialized nursing care and professional empowerment, seems most feasible. With this in mind, a voluntary system of governance (specialty review and approval), recognizing and involving existing interests, is herein proposed and described below.

Operating Premises

First of all, it must be acknowledged that, while it is the responsibility of the state to license for entry into nursing practice in order to safeguard the public, it is the responsibility of the profession to regulate its specialties as a means of recognizing and promoting advanced knowledge and skills and to ensure orderly development of the field.

State governments, third-party payers, accrediting agencies, employers, the public, and nurse specialists should be able to recognize and rely upon means established by the profession to designate and certify those demonstrating special competencies.

Nursing's voluntary system for regulating specialties should not compete with the multiple functions of general or specialty organizations. It should recognize the national voluntary certification of specialists as the critical mechanism for bringing quality control to specialty practice and unity, homogeneity, and authority to the development of specialties.

Thus the voluntary governance system proposed herein should serve the single purpose of reviewing and approving specialties and their standards and processes of certification and accreditation.

The approved specialties may, in turn, conduct, delegate, recognize, or contract for certification and accreditation programs.

For purposes of further discussion, this voluntary governance mechanism will be referred to as the National Board of Nursing Specialties, abbreviated as the Board or NBNS. This Board should meet several specifications.

1. The NBNS should be based upon the principle of voluntary approval of specialties. For reasons related to quality of services and enhancement of the profession and the specialty and its members, specialties may choose to be reviewed by the Board, to be designated as Board-approved, and to have their specialists certified by an NBSN-approved certifying body.

2. The Board should be based upon a system of peer review combined with professional and public oversight. Specialties, as a body, would review and approve one another, initially and periodically, according to standards developed jointly with the profession-at-large and in a way that provides for public consultation.

3. The structure and function of the Board should provide for representation of the specialties themselves, the profession-at-large, and the public interests. The degree and nature of participation within the various structures and relationships of the Board would be based upon equity, purpose, and function. For example, policy-making, standard-setting, and the review process would require different arenas and modes of participation. Therefore, the policy-making body should include broad representation from all sectors of the profession, from the specialties as a whole, and the lay public. The review bodies should include representatives from approved specialty boards.

4. The Board should maintain explicit ties to the total profession and should both shape and defer to the good interests of the profession as a whole.

5. The Board should be self-sustaining and have adequate resources to conduct its critical and singular function of reviewing and approving specialties and their standards and processes of certification and accreditation.

6. The approval and review process of the Board should be based upon explicit criteria and should provide an appeals process.

7. Because of the current diversity in specialist certification, a transition plan should be developed to enable specialties to meet standards and criteria within a reasonable time period.

Appendix C-1 (p. 178) outlines a prototype of a board of nursing specialties embracing the above premises and principles.

Criteria for Approval of Specialties

What criteria would be most appropriate for such a board to use in reviewing specialties to determine their adequacy of standard and fit? This question brings us to the second set of recommendations. Important resources in developing the following proposed criteria were documents produced by the California Nurses Association (1984), the Canadian Nurses Association (1985), the International Council of Nurses Professional Services Committee (1987), the American Board of Medical Specialties (1987), and the American Pharmaceutical Association's Board of Pharmaceutical Specialties (1975).

As subsystems of nursing, specialties should individually demonstrate the viability and effectiveness of their functional components (practice, education, research, peer review/credentialing) and should in the aggregate evidence a high degree of homogeneity among themselves and a high degree of fit within the total profession. With these objectives in mind, the following criteria are proposed for use by a national board of nursing specialties in reviewing specialties applying for approval. An approved specialty should present evidence that:

1. The specialty defines itself as nursing and subscribes to the overall purpose and functions of nursing.
2. The specialty subscribes to the overall education, practice, and ethical standards of the profession.
3. There is both demand and need for the services of the specialty.
4. The specialty is national in its geographic scope.
5. The specialty is clearly defined in relationship to and differentiated from other specialties.
6. The specialty is sufficiently complex and advanced that it is beyond the qualifications for general practice.
7. Practice standards have been developed for the specialty.
8. The specialty knowledge base is well developed and is concerned with phenomena and problems within the discipline and practice of nursing.
9. Mechanisms exist for supporting, reviewing, and disseminating research.
10. Advanced education programs, leading to a certificate or graduate degree in nursing, prepare specialists in the field. A process exists for peer review of such programs to ensure that the standards of the Board are met.
11. The area of specialization includes a substantial number of practitioners who devote most of their practice to the specialty.
12. Practitioners of the specialty are licensed as registered nurses.
13. A peer review certification program exists to evaluate candidates to ensure initial and continued competence in the specialty.
14. Practitioners are organized and represented within a specialty association or branch of a parent organization.

Operational criterion measures would need to be applied to the above criteria.

Several of the criteria are concerned with the specialties' fit with one another and within the total field of nursing. This suggests the need for an overall pattern or, at least, some general guidelines for the organization of nursing's subsystems.

Thus is proffered the third set of recommendations regarding a specialization schema.

A Specialization Schema

Chapter III on the characteristics of nursing specialties today examined nursing's divisions of knowledge and practice as evidenced in specialty organizations, state and national certification or recognition programs, graduate programs in nursing, etc. It was determined that specialties have organized around (1) roles, (2) loci or systems of care, (3) developmental stages of care recipients, (4) anatomical or functional systems or processes, (5) diseases or pathology, and (6) technologies or treatment modalities. Is there some way of guiding nursing's development into a more rational, more comprehensive, less duplicative, functional pattern of specialties, subspecialties, and related certification programs?

First of all, what is nursing? The ANA, in *Nursing: A Social Policy Statement*, has defined nursing as "the diagnosis and treatment of human responses to actual or potential health problems" (ANA, 1980, p. 9). The International Council of Nurses (ICN), in adopting the 1985 position paper on the regulation of nursing worldwide (ICN, 1985), committed itself to defining specialization and identifying the major "branches" of nursing practice. Accordingly, the Professional Services Committee (PSC) of the ICN has developed a draft statement on specialization, proposing six "major branches" of nursing (medical/surgical nursing, maternal-child health nursing, pediatric nursing, geriatric nursing, mental health/psychiatric nursing, and public health/community nursing). These branches have been more or less recognized historically and internationally, although they are often disparaged as representing a "medical model." The proposal under review within ICN went on to endorse the concept of branching, i.e., specialties and subspecialties, acknowledging that certain specialties may originate from more than one major branch of the field. For example, pediatric oncology could arise from the nursing of children or from cancer nursing (PSC, 1987).

Medicine, the field most analogous to nursing in scope and complexity, if not orientation and phenomena, has acknowledged that boundaries between specialties are often "hazy and overlapping" (ABMS, 1983, p. 47), and that specialties "may entail concern with the problems of patients according to age, sex, or organ systems or with the interaction between patients and their environment" (ABMS, 1983, p. 83).

In dealing with these variables, the medical profession has evolved a system of 23 specialty boards, each offering a general certification and from 1 to 10 "special certifications," yielding a total of more than 60 areas of specialty practice. Subspecialists must first qualify in the specialty (ABMS, 1987). Appendix C-2 (p. 181) outlines the categories of medical certification. Most of the member boards are primary; a small number are conjoint, reflecting hybrid disciplines, e.g., the combining of pathology and radiology to create the fields of nuclear radiology and radioisotopic pathology. Obviously, medicine has chosen to negotiate and refine, rather than design, its specialties through the authoritative processes and criteria of the ABMS.

In view of nursing's already proliferative and somewhat random specialization (perhaps we should paraphrase from Teilhard de Chardin in the Prologue and describe nursing's development as "uncontrolled additivity"), the best route for the profession to take in attempting to derive some pattern for specialty development may be for the National Board of Nursing Specialties (NBNS) to develop a configuration of primary boards with certification programs fitting within those boards. It would have to be acknowledged from the outset that no perfect, trouble-free classification exists and that professional judgment will be an important factor in the application of criteria and categories. At the time of applying for review, specialties would probably be asked to declare and justify their perceived best fit.

A number of schemata could be considered. Four possibilities are listed below. For purposes of discussion, the bi-level terms "primary and secondary boards," "board and certifications," and "specialty and subspecialty" are used permissively and interchangeably to differentiate between the broad practice categories and the specialty clusters within.

Schema A (by clinical branches and specialties)

Under this schema, depicted in Figure 2, boards would correspond approximately to the clinical branches identified by the ICN—medical-surgical, maternal-child health, pediatric, geriatric, mental health/psychiatric, and public health/community nursing. Specialties would fit within these boards. Subspecialties would fit within the specialties. Bi-level certification programs could be accommodated within a specialty. Were such a configuration to be adopted, a number of observations, challenges, and questions would have to be addressed:

1. The broadest areas of certification today, i.e., the clinical branches identified by ICN, are represented within the generalist certification programs of the ANA.
2. Would specialists be expected to qualify in the primary branch before proceeding to secondary certification? In other words, would the relationship of branch to specialty be encompassing and sequential or segregated?

FIGURE 2 Boards Corresponding to Clinical Branches

Boards

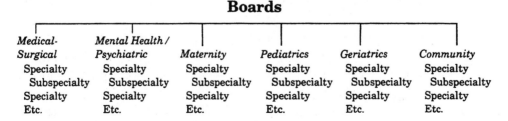

Medical-Surgical	Mental Health/Psychiatric	Maternity	Pediatrics	Geriatrics	Community
Specialty	Specialty	Specialty	Specialty	Specialty	Specialty
Subspecialty	Subspecialty	Subspecialty	Subspecialty	Subspecialty	Subspecialty
Specialty	Specialty	Specialty	Specialty	Specialty	Specialty
Etc.	Etc.	Etc.	Etc.	Etc.	Etc.

3. What standards, educational and otherwise, would apply to the primary certification vis-a-vis the more specialized certification?
4. How would a specialty schema of specialties and subspecialties relate to graduate programs in nursing? Would such programs be designed to prepare for the primary or secondary specialty or both?
5. Where would functional specialties, such as administration, consultation, etc., fit within such a configuration?

Schema B (by roles or categories of specialists)

Under this schema, depicted in Figure 3, boards would correspond to categories of specialists—e.g., generalist certifications (the broader branches of clinical nursing), clinical nurse specialty certifications, nurse practitioner certifications, functional specialty certifications. Various categories of specialists could include subspecialties or bi-level certification programs. Such a schema might force a distinction between clinical nurse specialists and nurse practitioners, or it could perpetuate the current confusion.

Other schemata

Other schemata of boards and certifications could be designed around other variables that have not occurred to the author or have been viewed as too problematic.

No schema

It would also be possible to operate with no configuration of boards and certifications, i.e., in a unidivisional manner with all specialties and certification programs being lodged within and reviewed by a single body. Difficulties presented would be these:

1. The span of responsibility and peer review would be as broad as the profession.
2. Variables defining specialization could continue to proliferate and the conceptualization of nursing practice could become more diffuse.
3. Competition and duplication among specialties could worsen.
4. Operationalization of the concept of specialties and subspecialties could be retarded.

FIGURE 3 Boards Corresponding to Categories of Specialists

Boards

Generalist Certifications	Clinical Specialist Certifications	Nurse Practitioner Certifications	Functional Certifications
1	1	1	1
2	2	2	2
Etc.	Etc.	Etc.	Etc.

Although the flexibility and diplomacy of the profession's leadership will be taxed to achieve agreement in such a major developmental task, it must be accomplished. Overall it would be difficult, if not impossible, to advance the goal of unity of fit among nursing's specialty subsystems without such a schema. The schema chosen must relate most closely to the realities of practice and the clusters of knowledge and skill needed to fulfill evolving practice roles. Therefore, it would seem unwise and impractical to consider those theoretical formulations and nursing diagnosis taxonomies—so essential for other purposes—as a framework for organizing specialties.

Transition Plan

Need for a Transition Plan

If certification is to play its full role in professionalizing nursing, standards for specialty certification must be high. There are several reasons for believing that a fitting *goal* for educational preparation for specialty certification would be a graduate degree in nursing added to the BSN generalist base:

- Trends in nursing education indicate an increased proportion of RNs holding a minimum of a BSN degree.
- The Tri-Council for Nursing (American Association of Colleges of Nursing, American Nurses' Association, American Organization of Nurse Executives, and the National League for Nursing) and many specialty organizations have accepted the BSN as the minimum preparation for the generalist professional nurse of the future.
- A specialist program and degree would appropriately be positioned at the next higher level above the generalist base in the academic hierarchy.
- The majority of nurses surveyed in our convenience sample favored the master's degree as the educational standard for specialty practice certification (Appendix B-2, p. 169).

While the goal of graduate degree preparation for nurse specialists seems both proper and ultimately feasible, contemporary *realities* must be faced:

- The majority of nurse specialists today are not graduate-prepared in areas of specialization.
- Very few of the national specialties currently require this educational credential for certification; some others plan to move toward such a standard.
- The number of BSN-prepared recruits is not adequate to fill the immediate need for certified specialists.
- The master's degree programs in nursing may not be adequate in number, quality, and focus to provide the graduate education appropriate to some specialties. Graduate-prepared, certified specialist faculty are a limited resource.

In view of this gap between tomorrow's *goal* and today's *realities,* it seems essential that an acceptable *transition plan* be developed if the proposal for the National Board of Nursing Specialties (NBNS), setting high standards for certification, is to gain the support and participation of specialty groups. It would be the responsibility of the NBNS to develop and approve such a plan for its members, considering a number of factors such as those indicated below.

Factors to Be Considered

The following factors should be considered in the elaboration of a transition plan for raising the educational requirements for specialty certification.

1. **Degree of conformity to standard and degree of conformity to timetable.** How much uniformity among specialties is desirable and feasible in conforming to the transition plan, its standards, and its timetable? As to timetable, two options may be identified:
   a. All member specialties would have to implement the accepted minimum standard by an agreed-upon date, or
   b. Member specialties would only be required to submit an acceptable plan and timetable, i.e., implementation dates may vary.

   As to conformity to standards, although there are discrepancies throughout certification processes and requirements, the greatest disparity is likely to be with respect to the educational credential. Must all specialties conform to the highest level set by NBNS from options indicated below?

2. **Objectives.** What are interim and ultimate objectives with respect to minimum education requirements for specialty certification? For example, five options, in descending order, are:
   a. BSN base + MSN minimum in the specialty
   b. BSN base + MSN or equivalent in the specialty
   c. BSN base or equivalent + MSN or equivalent in the specialty
   d. BSN base + certificate program of specified nature and length in the specialty
   e. BSN or equivalent base + certificate program of specified nature and length in the specialty

   What requirements must the educational programs meet to be accepted/accredited for certification purposes? For example:
   a. Degree programs offered in NLN-accredited schools of nursing
   b. Non-degree certificate programs approved by ANA and/or by the specialty itself
   c. Other specific requirements set by the NBNS

3. **Timetable.** What is the year or juncture at which the ultimate objective is to be achieved? For example, might the specialty preparation objective be tied to the point at which a certain percentage of RNs are BSN-prepared? Moreover, might the objectives be reached in a phased manner, for example, BSN base at one point, BSN base + MSN in the specialty at a later date? And, as

indicated above, must the timetable for all specialties be congruent? Similarly, will dates for implementation of approval/accreditation of educational programs be uniform?

4. **Interim arrangements.** What arrangements are possible and necessary during the transition to avoid jeopardizing currently certified nurses and the availability of specialists to meet practice needs? Some options are:

    a. Establishment of bi-level certification programs, with the intention of progressing solely to the higher standard

    b. Indefinite grandfathering[2] of individuals certified prior to a certain date, as long as they continue to meet testing and/or practice requirements for recertification

    c. Grandfathering[2] for a specified period, allowing currently certified nurses the time to upgrade their educational qualifications

    d. Adoption of evaluation procedures to assess equivalency for those who do not meet the education standard

5. **Certification program development.** What consultation and resources are necessary to assist specialties to refine and improve certification processes and procedures and to implement their transition plans? What government and/or private funds would be available to facilitate this development?

6. **Educational program development.** What incentives would encourage schools to develop graduate curricula to match specialty preparation needs? How could the AACN and NLN contribute to this development? What resources are necessary? What governmental and private resources could be made available?

Initial Steps

These proposals represent two phases or processes for empowering nursing and its specialties. The first phase has to do with strengthening the specialties and their credentials. The second has to do with promoting or marketing the specialties and their credentials in those sectors now relatively immune to the latent power of the specialization movement in nursing.

Phase One:
Strengthening Specialty Credentials

Three initial steps are proposed to implement phase one of this proposal, i.e., the enhancement of specialty credentials through the creation of the National Board of Nursing Specialties established to review and approve specialties and their certification programs.

---

2. *Grandfathering* refers to creating an exemption based upon pre-existing standards.

A consensus conference, made up of representatives of the organizations that are the prospective regular and associate members of the NBNS, should be held to study and refine this proposal and set into motion its implementation. In preparation for this meeting, a technical and strategic advisory committee should develop the strategy for the conference and further develop the proposal for the NBNS. (See Prototype for NBNS in Appendix C-1, p. 178.)

A resource development task force, made up of representatives of private and governmental funding sources and the nursing education and specialty sectors, should identify needs for educational and certification program development (Transition Plan, Factors 5 and 6) and devise a comprehensive strategy to address those needs. The proposal for the NBNS should be greatly reinforced by evidence of resources to assist in these areas.

An Interim Board or Committee should be established after the consensus conference to include representatives from the currently existing specialty boards and other organizations with a stake in the development of specialty nursing practice. The Interim Board or Committee would draw up articles of incorporation, bylaws, dues assessments, policies, standards, criteria and mechanisms for reviewing specialty certifying boards, and procedures for electing officers and trustees. The Interim Board or Committee would have to deal initially with fundamental questions, such as:

▮ The appropriate configuration of boards and certifications, i.e., branches/ specialties and subspecialties,
▮ Distinctions between generalists practicing in a specialty, clinical nurse specialists, nurse practitioners, etc., in titling, standards, and certifications, and
▮ The place of functional vis-a-vis clinical specialties.

Throughout this process it would be essential for the Interim Board or Committee to communicate and consult with potential constituencies.

Interim status of the Board or Committee and its specialty members would continue until such time as initial reviews had been conducted and regular members admitted. A category might be created for provisional members who aspire to but do not yet meet standards for approval as Board-certified specialties and as regular members of the NBNS.

Phase Two:
Promoting Specialty Credentials

As a corollary process, the marketing or promotion of specialty credentials, strengthened through the above process, should occur.

Information about the NBNS and its certifications should be circulated. A complete registry of certificate holders should be maintained. Recognition of specialty credentials must be systematically and forcefully promoted in the following sectors, using all possible sources of influence:

- Career-oriented nurses,
- Health care accreditation standards, federal and state,
- Public awareness,
- Salary and career advancement,
- Regulatory arenas, federal and state,
- Third-party reimbursement mechanisms, public and private, federal and state,
- Employment standards, job descriptions,
- Health agency recruitment,
- Nursing school faculty standards,
- Development of graduate curricula,
- Research and project grant applications,
- Media portrayal of nursing,
- Health care consumers, and
- Recruitment into nursing.

This developmental work should begin immediately because there is much progress to be made and because such a "marketing" plan should stimulate interest in and support for the formation of an NBNS. Standardizing and strengthening the certification credential, giving it a powerful and common meaning, must be seen as essential to the promotion of the credential. Philanthropic and professional resources and responsibilities should be identified for various aspects of the promotion plan.

Closing

This monograph ends as it began in the Preface with "the burning desire to empower nursing to achieve its eminent destiny in the public interest." It is hoped that this analysis of nursing specialization and the ensuing proposals for a new empowerment will be well considered by the profession.

May the reader and all those in positions of influence share the author's vision that through self-regulation nursing shall become—

- As strong as it is noble,
- As magnetic as it is meritorious,
- As powerful as it is important,
- As professional as it is humane,
- As unified as it is dedicated,

and that we shall take control where we now have permission.

References

Accreditation Council for Graduate Medical Education (ACGME, 1987). *1987–1988 directory of graduate medical education programs.* Chicago, IL: American Medical Association.

American Board of Medical Specialties (ABMS, 1987). *ABMS compendium supplement.* Evanston, IL: Author.

American Board of Medical Specialties (ABMS, 1983). *Annual report and reference handbook 1983.* Evanston, IL: Author.

American Dental Association (ADA, 1986). *Handbook for predental advisors.* Chicago: Author.

American Dental Association (ADA, 1982, December). *Requirements for advanced specialty education programs.* Chicago, IL: Author.

American Pharmaceutical Association (APhA, 1975). Criteria Adopted by APhA for Recognition of Specialties in Pharmacy Practice. Unpublished document.

American Nurses' Association (ANA, 1979). *The study of credentialing in nursing: A new approach.* Kansas City, MO: Author.

American Nurses' Association (ANA, 1980). *Nursing: A social policy statement.* Kansas City, MO: Author.

California Nurses Association (1984). *Position statement on specialization in nursing practice.* San Francisco: Author.

Call, R. L. (1987). The impact of required postdoctoral programs on predoctoral and specialty education. *The Journal of Dental Education, 51(6),* 298–301.

Canadian Nurses Association (1985). *Policy statement on credentialing in nursing.* Report of the Canadian Nurses Association Ad Hoc Committee on Credentialing.

International Council of Nurses (1985). *Report on the regulation of nursing.* Geneva: Author.

Penna, R. (1988). Private communication with author.

Professional Services Committee (PSC), International Council of Nurses (1987). Specialization in Nursing Discussion Document 1987. (Unpublished.)

Walton, C. A. (1986). Specialization in pharmacy practice. *Drug Intelligence and Clinical Pharmacy, 20,* 279–280.

Zellmer, W. A. (1986). Specialization (Editorial). *American Journal of Hospital Pharmacy, 49, 1191.*

Index